Breathing N

Adenoids Without Surgery

Avoid Adenoidectomy Naturally
Breathing Exercises and Lifestyle
Recommendations
For Children and Parents

Illustrated Guide for Parents

Written by
Sasha Yakovleva

Afterword by Ira Packman, MD
Illustrations by Arash Akhgari

Adenoids Without Surgery
Copyright © 2015 Alexandra Yakovleva
BreathingCenter Publications

www.BreathingCenter.com

info@breathingcenter.com

ISBN: 978-1984940827

Printed in the USA

All rights reserved. No part of this book may be reproduced or utilized in any form or by any means, including photographs, recordings, or by any information storage or retrieval system or technologies now known or later developed, electronic or mechanical, without permission in writing from the Publisher.

Illustrations: Arash Akhgari

Afterword: Ira Packman, MD

Text: Sasha Yakovleva

Afterword: Ira Packman, MD

Editing: Ethan Campbell, Tusha Yakovleva, Cole Larsen
Final editing: Jean Boles

Front cover illustration: Arash Akhgari
Back cover illustration: Arash Akhgari

Cover and interior design: Jean Boles
www.jean.bolesbooks@gmail.com

Dedication

*This book is dedicated to my teachers,
Ludmila Buteyko and Andrey Novozhilov, MD.*

*Special thanks to Ethan Campbell
for his help in creating this book.*

Contents

Chapter One: The Purpose of This Book 9
Chapter Two: Breathing Normalization and Children with Enlarged Adenoids 14
Chapter Three: Enlarged Adenoids Without Surgery 19
Chapter Four: Testimonials 27
Chapter Five: Breathing and its Measurements 31
    Over-Breathing 31
    Healthy Breathing 32
    Close Your Mouth 33
    Why Does My Child Hyperventilate? 35
    Breathing Measurements 36
    How To Take Breathing Measurements 37
    When To Take Breathing Measurements 40
    How To Record Breathing Measurements 41
    How To Read Breathing Measurements 41
        The Norm: 43
        1st Level of Hyperventilation: 43
        2nd Level of Hyperventilation: 43
        3rd Level of Hyperventilation: 44
        4th Level of Hyperventilation: 44
        5th Level of Hyperventilation: 44
        The Last Line Of The Chart: 44

    Healing Crisis 46

    How To Recognize The Healing Crisis 47

Chapter Six: Lifestyle Recommendations 48

    Stress Reduction 48

    Breathing During Sleep 50

        Tape: 51

        Scarf: 52

        Other factors: 53

    Physical Activity 53

    Diet 57

        What to drink: 57

        What to Eat: 57

        Hunger: 58

        Salt: 59

    Nature 59

    Talking 61

Chapter Seven: Breathing Exercises for Children 63

    I. Breathing Exercises in a Still Position: 68

        Do I Breathe Through my Mouth? 68

        1. American Indian Mother 69

        2. Show Me Your Breathing 71

        3. Is my Breathing Noisy? 72

        4. Are my Shoulders/Chest/Stomach Moving? 72

        5. Book on the Belly 74

        6. Hug a Tree 75

        7. A Little Mouse 76

    8. Be a Samurai 77

    9. Tape Exercises 78

    10. Nose Songs 80

    11. Polly's Angel 81

    12. A Sophisticated Device 82

    13. Fixed Breath Holds 83

    14. Flexible Breath Holds 84

II. Breathing Exercises in Motion 85

    15. Dancing with a Nose Song 85

    16. Airplane 86

    17. Walking, Hiking, Running 87

        ~ Walking 87

        ~ Hiking 88

        ~ Running 88

    18. A Corner-to-Corner Walk with Breath Holds 89

    19. Don't Miss the Fridge 90

    20. Steps with Breath Holds 91

    21. Walk with Breath Holds 92

    22. Simple Jumps 93

    23. Three-Fold Jumps 94

        ~ Jumping: 94

        ~ Running: 95

        ~ Walking: 95

III. Breathing Exercises for Relaxation 97

    24. Imagine 98

    25. I am Not a Robot 99

  26. Heating Pad 100

  27. Tense Up 101

 IV. Breathing Exercises to Stop Symptoms 102

  28. Nodding 102

  29. The Breathing Guru 103

  30. Coughing 104

Chapter Eight: Peter's Mom's Journal 105

Chapter Nine: Questions and Answers 115

Chapter Ten: One More Testimonial 121

Breathing Logbook 129

Afterword: By Ira J Packman, MD 133

About the Author and Contributors 138

Past

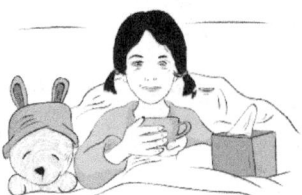

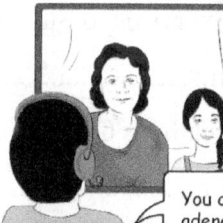
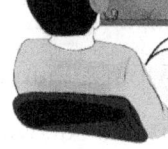
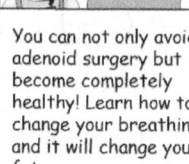
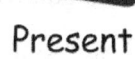

Present

You can not only avoid adenoid surgery but become completely healthy! Learn how to change your breathing and it will change your future.

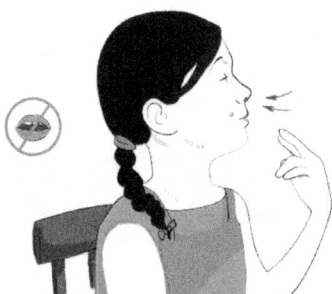

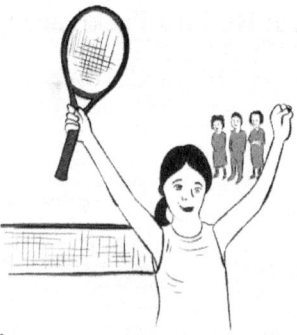

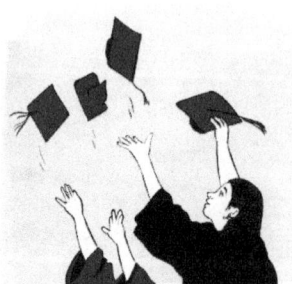

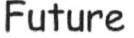

Future

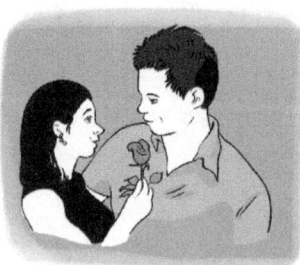

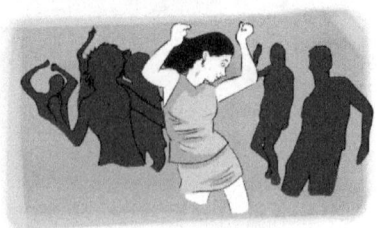

Chapter One

The Purpose of This Book

At the start of the week, I had a Preliminary Consultation via an online video call with a 15-year-old girl suffering from enlarged adenoids. She attended the consultation from home with her mother and aunt, both of whom were very concerned about Annie's health.

Annie was strikingly beautiful—like a little flower ready to bloom. However, her voice was terribly coarse as a result of taking steroids and other medication. She quickly ran out of breath and her breathing was forceful and loud. Her voice clearly indicated her poor health.

Annie's mother shared that her daughter had two adenoid removal surgeries and was awaiting the third, since her adenoids were growing back again. Normally, adenoids atrophy when a child is around twelve years old, but Annie's would not give up. Her tonsils had been removed a few years ago. Her energy level was low but she was often overly excited and sometimes had trouble concentrating. Her nose was often runny or stuffy, and every winter, she would miss many school days due to frequent colds and flu. When spring and summer came, Annie had a pollen allergy. She used a rescue inhaler periodically; Annie's doctor warned her parents that their daughter was developing asthma.

Being a mother of a daughter myself, I immediately felt a strong wave of compassion toward Annie. I thought, *I wish she had taken our Breathing Normalization program years ago.* All her trouble could have been stopped then! So, what does her future look like now? Soon, this teenager will start dating… will others be able to see the flower I saw before I witnessed her illness. Soon, she will start thinking about college. With low energy and difficulty concentrating, her chances are slim! Later in life, if she becomes a mother, there is no way for her children to be healthy since they inherit her breathing patterns! Annie is going to be unnecessarily hampered by a treatable illness!

Instead of sharing those thoughts, I only said, "The Breathing Center can help Annie. Our individual Breathing Normalization program will stop her adenoids from growing further and will eliminate the necessity for an adenoidectomy. It will end all her respiratory trouble."

For Annie's mother and aunt, this sounded almost too good to be true. They told me that they had already tried many alternative therapies but to no avail. I was not surprised: many parents spend a lot of time and money trying everything before they are lucky enough to find the Breathing Normalization method, which finally puts an end to their children's respiratory troubles. Being skeptical, both women started bombarding me with questions, which I was eager to answer. Their questions were informed and also interesting because they came from two radically different perspectives. Annie's mother was a pharmacist, while her aunt was a yoga teacher. Since the Breathing Normalization method does not conflict with either of these modalities and even unites them, my answers satisfied both women.

Annie's story also resonated with personal experiences the two women had. Apparently, both sisters had been suffering from asthma their entire lives. Everything I told them about mouth-breathing and over-breathing as a cause of various breathing maladies, including adenoid growth as well as asthma, made sense to them.

I invited both sisters to participate in the Breathing Normalization program together with Annie. I told them, "During this breathing training, a Breathing Normalization specialist will primarily work with Annie; however, by following this method, both of you will be able to reduce or even stop your breathing difficulties."

While everyone was enthusiastic about the program, Annie's mother was concerned about the price of a two-month training; however, we arranged a payment plan, which made it affordable for the family. Since they lived in Hungary, we decided to conduct the program online. They liked the fact that there was no need to travel to the United States where Breathing Center is located. The training was fully available from their home via Skype, an online video-calling program, which would save them not only time but also money.

"When can we start?" Annie's mother asked me impatiently.

"Annie does not have any time to waste," I answered. "I suggest we start the program as soon as possible." Annie's mother assured me that they would sign up for the course right away, as soon as she discussed it with her husband.

A week passed and I still had not heard anything about Annie. This girl touched my heart and I kept thinking about her. Eventually, I called Annie's mother to find out the reason for this delay.

"After talking to my husband, we changed our plan," she explained. "Instead of Breathing Normalization, we decided to try homeopathy. My husband wants to give it a try for a year or so; if it does not work, he would reconsider. It's less expensive, you know! Besides, he does not believe that breathing improvement is effective, especially through the Internet!"

I admire homeopathy as well as many other holistic modalities, but in my experience, it does not prevent adenoidectomy or stop all respiratory trouble. Unless the breathing patterns are brought back to their natural rhythm by working with the breathing directly, a child with Annie's problems cannot be restored back to full health.

Annie's father was wrong, but it was not my place to argue. I said goodbye to Annie's mother and wished the family all the best.

Sasha Yakovleva

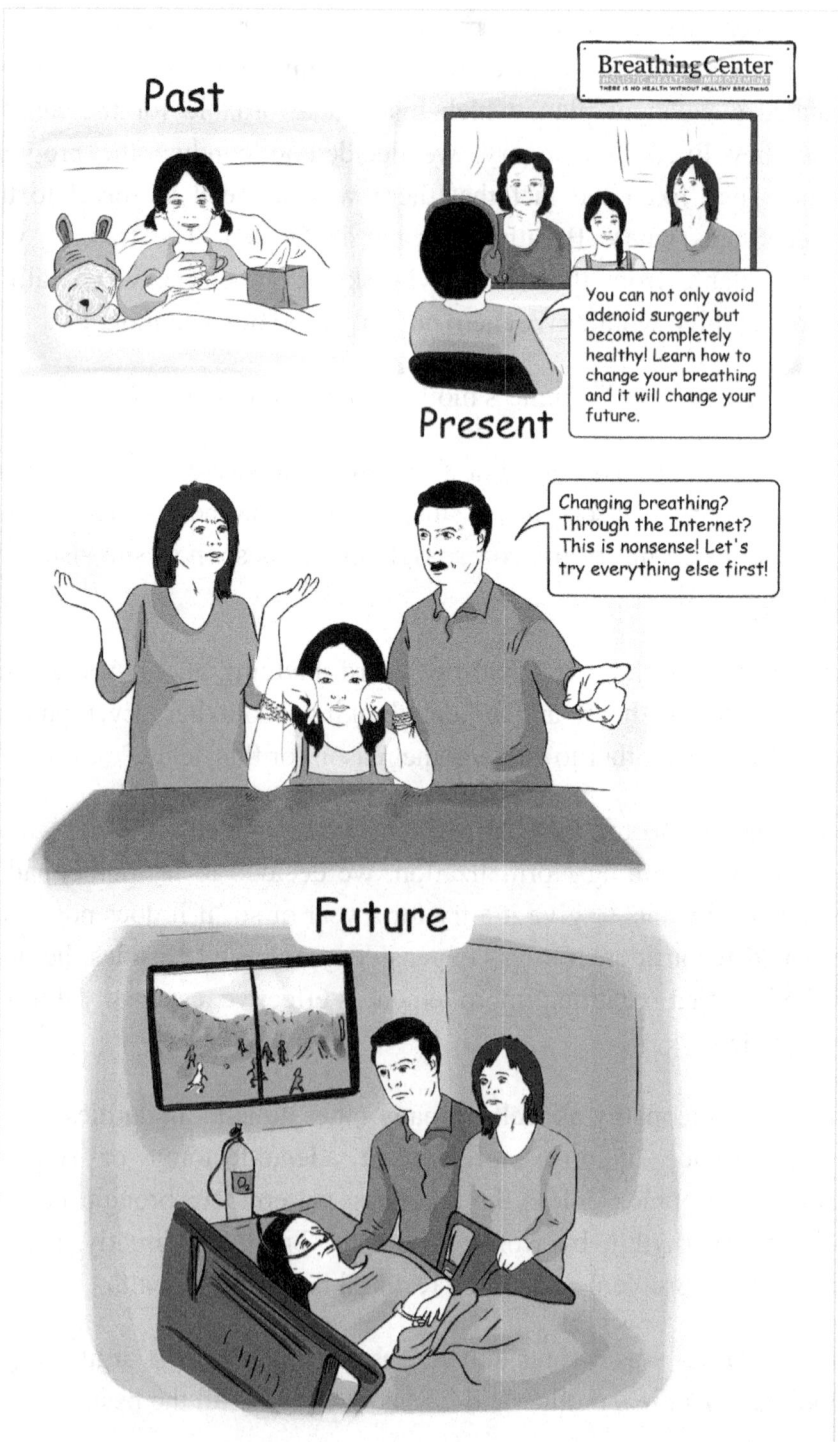

Obviously, not every Preliminary Consultation results in participation in our course. It happens periodically for various reasons: some parents lack the time, finances or commitment to help their children. I always feel sorry for children with enlarged adenoids who aren't given a chance to improve their breathing. Instead, they end up under the surgeon's knife, having an important part of their immune system removed.

As we know, there is always some risk with surgeries—in rare cases, children die from an adenoidectomy or tonsillectomy. Even a successful surgery can be physiologically and psychologically traumatic for a child. In addition, an adenoidectomy is not the solution to a child's long-term health issues. It provides a temporary fix, while its long-term effect can worsen the child's health and lead to further development of respiratory issues such as bronchitis, coughing, allergies, asthma, sleep apnea and other health problems.

This book is written with the single purpose: to give parents a chance to strengthen their child's health and change their child's destiny. It is a simple, step-by-step guide on how to avoid an adenoidectomy by naturally improving breathing and health. In this book, instructions are written for parents, grandparents or guardians, but the illustrations could be used by adults and kids, making breathing training more engaging and fun. For language clarity, I refer to a child as "he" throughout the book, but I am addressing children of all genders.

Yours in Health,
Sasha Yakovleva
Advanced Breathing Normalization Specialist
www.BreathingCenter.com

Chapter Two

Breathing Normalization and Children with Enlarged Adenoids

At the Breathing Center, we teach children and their parents how to normalize their breathing without medication and as an alternative to adenoid removal surgery. Our unique educational program, *Adenoid Without Surgery,* has been offered since 2009. During the six years it's been in existence, Breathing Normalization specialists have helped many children in the United States as well as other countries. We have worked with children from Nigeria, Mexico, New Zealand, Australia, Switzerland, Poland, Mexico, Ukraine, and other countries.

While the primary goal of the Breathing Normalization method is to correct breathing problems and restore normal breathing patterns, the method has a powerful effect on the health of one's entire body. The method is truly holistic: it improves the function of the whole body as one system without negative side effects. With consistent application of this method, not only are breathing difficulties eliminated, symptoms of many seemingly unrelated diseases are also reduced or disappear entirely.

This method is based on the discovery made by Konstantin Buteyko, MD, in Russia in 1952. His discovery was followed by more than 60 years of scientific and clinical work. The program—*Adenoid Without Surgery*—was created in 1987 by Andrey Novozhilov, MD, (who trained with and worked alongside Dr. Buteyko for decades) and a team of doctors at Clinica Buteyko™ Moscow. It was then carried over to the English-speaking world by Breathing Center—the exclusive representative of Clinica Buteyko Moscow. At the Breathing Center, the Buteyko Method was modified to fit a modern lifestyle and was renamed Breathing Normalization.

Breathing Normalization specialists certified by the Breathing Center are not medical doctors; however, they are trained by A. Novozhilov, MD, and other doctors. Together, Clinica Buteyko Moscow and Breathing Center in the U.S. have a great deal of experience helping children with enlarged adenoids.

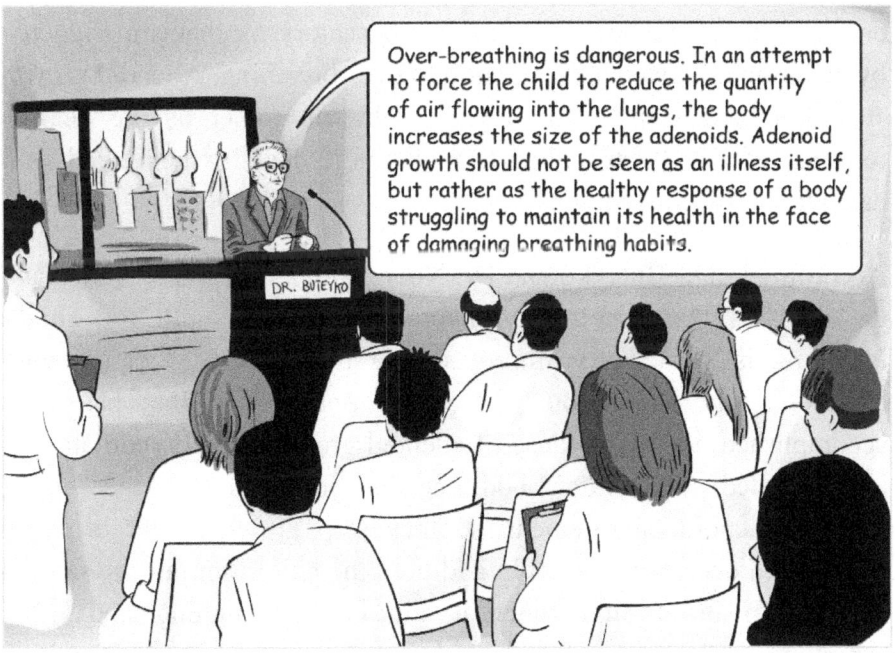

The key insight of the *Adenoids Without Surgery* program is that chronic over-breathing is the underlying cause of respiratory problems. In the case of enlarged adenoids, habitual mouth breathing as well as excessive breathing creates a very dangerous situation for the whole body. It causes edema and excess mucus as well as inflammation in the ears, nose, and throat area, increases probability of viral illnesses, and weakens the nervous system. In addition to this, the effects of hyperventilation create an oxygen deficiency in various organs (the Bohr effect) and disrupt normal metabolic functions. The result is that the child's immune system is suppressed, which leads to a broad range of health issues.

In an attempt to force the child to reduce the quantity of air flowing into the lungs (more precisely, being exchanged in the lungs; specifically, CO_2 being expelled) the body increases the size of the adenoids. It also increases mucus production, which partially coats the respiratory passages for this same reason—to restrict the passage of air, and thus, reduce hyperventilation. According to Dr. Buteyko, an enlargement of the adenoids is a compensatory mechanism triggered by the immune system as a reaction to over-breathing. Adenoid growth should not be seen as an illness itself, but rather as the healthy response of a body struggling to maintain its health when faced with damaging breathing habits.

According to Dr. Buteyko and Dr. Novozhilov, enlarged adenoids and the illnesses that accompany them will continue until the child's breathing is sufficiently improved. He must learn to consistently breathe gently and through the nose only. Once this has been accomplished, the main cause of adenoid growth—hyperventilation—is eliminated. The child's body no longer needs to protect itself through adenoid enlargement, so they stop growing, and in many cases, even decrease in size. In addition, the child's immune system is restored to its normal function and colds, coughing and other symptoms of enlarged adenoids go away. Since Breathing Normalization significantly improves the supply of oxygen to the brain and the other organs, children also become calmer and better able to concentrate. A strong immune system and better oxygen supply also prevents the development of other illnesses.

The restoration of a child's healthy breathing requires the full participation of at least one parent, but preferably the whole family.

Together with the child, a participating parent is present and active during every session with a Breathing Normalization specialist and works extensively with the child at home between sessions. No young child left alone is capable of the consistent application over an extended period of time that is necessary for effective treatment. Teenagers can do it alone; however, their progress is greatly accelerated by the support of their family.

The *Adenoid Without Surg*ery program contains two major elements: a change in lifestyle and breathing exercises. Since breathing patterns are the result of a lifestyle, it is essential for parents to modify their child's lifestyle to make it more conducive to healthy breathing. At the same time, a parent needs to ensure that a child practices breathing exercises to correct his unhealthy breathing habits. The majority of the breathing exercises are physical activities and games, so children usually experience them as entertainment.

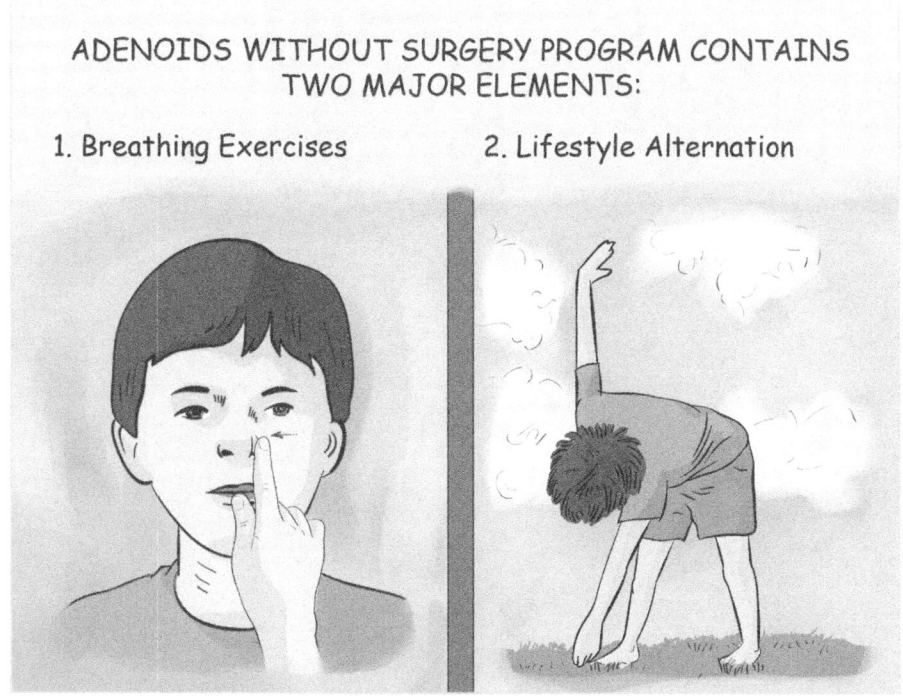

This book gives detailed instructions on both lifestyle changes and breathing exercises. It provides in-depth information in various forms: direct recommendations, a conversation with Dr. Novozhilov, stories about and from Breathing Center's clients and, drawings.

While we recommend working with a Breathing Normalization specialist directly when improving a child's breathing, I hope that the information in this book will make it possible for parents to help their child on their own. If you still have difficulties, you can contact the Breathing Center and schedule an online session with a specialist or take the Level 1 Breathing Normalization course. Working with a specialist remains the most comprehensive and effective approach!

Chapter Three

Enlarged Adenoids Without Surgery

*I*n 1999, I interviewed Doctor Novozhilov, Medical Director of Clinica Buteyko™ Moscow and the founder of the program, Adenoids Without Surgery. My conversation with him was published on Breathing Center's website. Since 1999, thousands of parents around the world have read it in their search for an alternative solution to help their children. In fact, this interview is the most visited page of Breathing Center's website. Here it is:

Sasha: *As a rule, children who have enlarged adenoids are plagued by colds, and their noses run constantly. In addition, they have periodic earaches. Sometimes, enlarged adenoids can lead to asthma. Is it really possible to alleviate these problems in children by removing the adenoids?*

Doctor Novozhilov: No, of course not. Surgical removal of the adenoids often improves a child's condition, but only in the beginning, sometimes for only a few weeks, after which the child begins to get sick again. Furthermore, it often turns out that the adenoids start to grow back after surgery. In one of our young patients, the adenoids were removed four times, and each time they came back again.

Sasha: *Then why do physicians recommend adenoid removal? They must be aware of the limited effectiveness of this operation.*

Doctor Novozhilov: Physicians certainly know that an adenoidectomy is not a panacea. However, in many cases, by temporarily improving a child's condition, it postpones the development of more serious illnesses. Aside from that, the physicians cannot offer anything. What else can be done to restore proper nasal breathing in a child? After all, the disruption of nasal breathing, ongoing nasal congestion, and the transition to breathing through the mouth are the very things that constitute the root of all evil in this instance. Steroids? Yes, they are able to eliminate the swelling of nasal mucus membranes, as well as restore one's ability to breathe through the nose, and this frequently proves to be a stepping-stone to a child's successful treatment. However, placing a child on hormones isn't the best idea. For this reason, physicians say: "It's better if we cut out the adenoids, especially since they might become inflamed."

Sasha: *Is the cause of adenoid growth known?*

Doctor Novozhilov: Mainstream medicine does not know the reason that adenoids grow, but in this regard, Professor Buteyko felt that adenoid growth is a defense mechanism of the body that is brought on by the disruption of the respiratory function. Have you ever noticed how a child with enlarged adenoids breathes? Usually, breathing in such a child is noisy, deep and through the mouth. This excessive respiration, or in other words "hyperventilation," is capable of inflicting tremendous damage to a child's body, since it causes oxygen starvation (the Verigo-Bohr effect), disrupts metabolism and impairs immunity. A child's body needs to protect itself against hyperventilation. It does this by blocking the respiratory canals by way of adenoid enlargement and the edema of the mucus membrane; that is to say, a chronic stuffy nose is unavoidable. When respiratory canals are constricted, the amount of air that a child exchanges in the lungs is reduced and, accordingly, the child's body does not sustain a high level of damage.

Sasha: *Which is to say that the cause of adenoid growth is hyperventilation. But can removing the adenoids actually halt hyperventilation?*

Doctor Novozhilov: No, never. That is why Professor Buteyko called adenoid removal surgery a crime against children. I also believe that, in most cases, the adenoids are removed in vain. Enlarged adenoids are nothing more than the body's defense mechanism against hyperventilation, and eliminating this defense reaction entails the development of more serious health problems. Other problems that also constitute a defense reaction frequently accompany enlarged adenoids—for example, a stuffy nose, a cough and so forth. If the adenoids are removed, hyperventilation persists; thus, these symptoms not only remain, but sometimes even intensify, since they have to take on the function previously performed by the adenoids. Removing the adenoids often leads to more serious defense reactions—for example, the child begins to experience bronchial spasms, which can ultimately lead to the development of asthma.

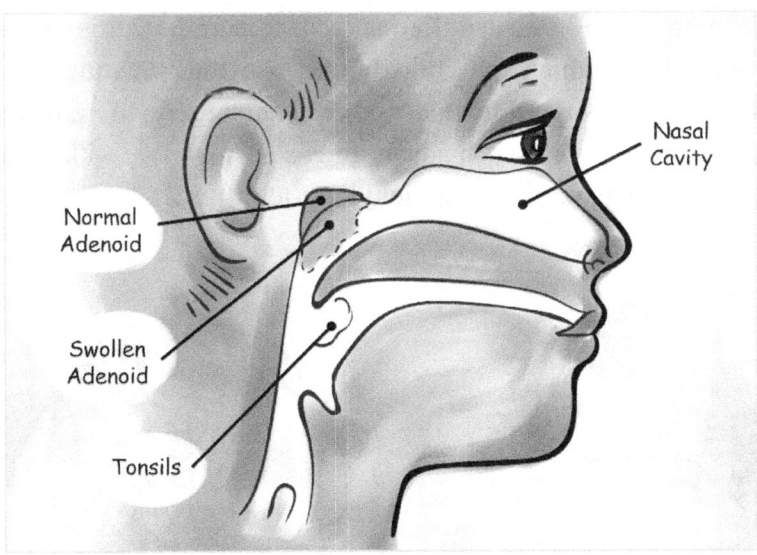

Sasha: *There is a prevailing belief that it is difficult for a child to breathe because his adenoids are enlarged, and that if they are cut out, it will then become easier for the child to breathe. But listening to you, it appears that exactly the opposite is true; it may be that it becomes even more difficult for the child to breathe after the adenoids are removed.*

Doctor Novozhilov: Yes, that is frequently what happens. In other cases, prolonged hyperventilation leads to a serious lowering of immunity and development of more serious illnesses.

Sasha: *And what would the result be if parents flatly refused surgery, but at the same time, did not follow Dr. Buteyko's approach?*

Doctor Novozhilov: More than likely, the lowering of immunity and development of new illnesses. As time goes by, if a child's nose becomes completely blocked and he is only able to breathe through the mouth, degradation may set in. The child's skull bones could become deformed; his face might change and be transformed into an "idiot face," in the medical sense of this term. Incidentally, the expression "adenoid face" even exists in medical circles. The adenoids may also become inflamed and infected; frequent ear infections (otitis) could set in, as a result of which the child might lose their hearing, at least partially. It is important to understand that surgery to remove the adenoids is imperative in such advanced cases; however, without using Dr. Buteyko's method, it cannot yield long-term results.

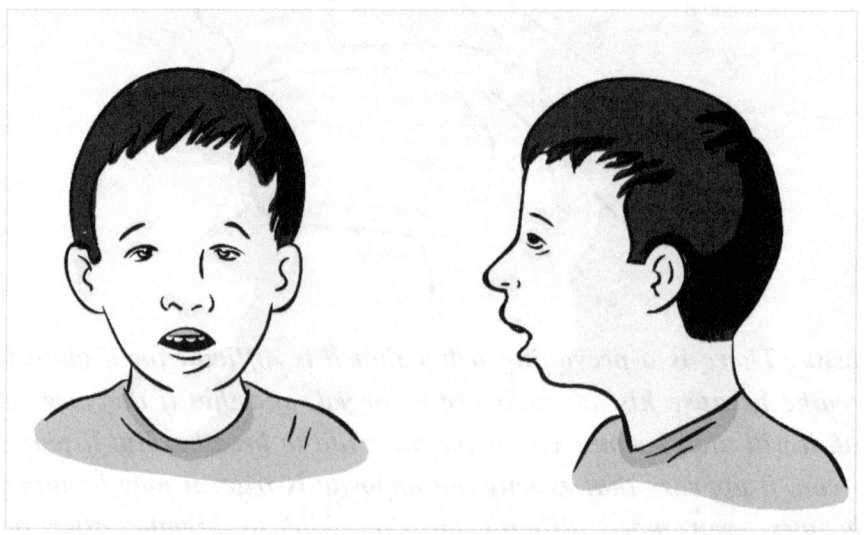

Sasha: *Okay, but what would Buteyko breathing specialists be able to propose in the event of enlarged adenoids?*

Doctor Novozhilov: We approach this problem in a different way. The cause of enlarged adenoids is hyperventilation; consequently, it is necessary to eliminate the cause of the illness, then its symptoms will go away on their own. The primary objective of a specialist is to normalize a child's breathing, first and foremost, by restoring breathing through the nose. A child who is not able to breathe through the nose will never be healthy.

Sasha: *That's easy to say—to restore breathing through the nose! But after all, a child with enlarged adenoids is scarcely able to breathe through the nose.*

Doctor Novozhilov: You are right, Sasha. The restoration of nasal breathing in a child is quite a difficult task, and therefore it must be accomplished under the supervision of a specialist. Indeed, it is hard for a child with enlarged adenoids to breathe through the nose. This is true for two reasons: on the one hand, adenoids block the flow of air through the nose; while on the other hand, it is blocked by the swelling of mucus membrane in the nose. Edema severely constricts the respiratory passages and can ultimately cover the adenoids themselves, at which point the nose ceases breathing altogether. That is to say, the problem consists of two parts: enlarged adenoids, which cannot be reduced in most cases once they grow, and edema of the mucosa, which can be reduced. If the edema goes away, a child will once again be able to breathe through the nose, while the adenoids themselves atrophy when the child reaches age twelve.

Sasha: *But what happens if the edema does not go away?*

Doctor Novozhilov: As a result of edema, normal air circulation of the nasopharynx (ears, nose, and throat area) is impaired, and so is natural fluid drainage (discharge). As a result of this, the adenoids become inflamed, and if microbes enter the picture, pus is produced. Edema starts to spread, gradually engulfing the entire ear, nose and throat area and affects the ventilation openings of the ears. When edema covers these openings, inner ear inflammation then sets in, frequently accompanied by hearing loss. But this is not a true deafness; the child is in a condition such that his ears are "stuffed up," as is the case, for example, in an airplane. Eliminating the mucosal edema through breathing exercises often prompts children to say that their "hearing has returned." To the parents, this usually sounds like a "miracle cure." But, it has to be wistfully observed that parents, through lack of knowledge, often take their child to a physician, and a surgeon cuts out their inflamed adenoids. Consequently, a sort of "hole" is shaped within the nose and it becomes easier for the child to breathe. However, the edema is still there; in a certain amount of time, it will again cover this hole and the child's nose will again be clogged. History repeats itself! Edema also makes it very difficult for a surgeon to cut out the adenoids completely, as a consequence of which, a small piece of tissue is occasionally left behind and it re-grows. Therefore, in six months or so, the child often has to face adenoid removal again.

Sasha: *So, it turns out that the most important thing for the successful treatment of a child with enlarged adenoids is to eliminate the swelling of mucus membrane.*

Doctor Novozhilov: That's exactly right!

Sasha: *And how is this done?*

Doctor Novozhilov: There are two ways. One of them is the use of steroids, which ultimately inflict considerable damage on a child's health. But the second method is safe and does not have any adverse consequences—that is to get rid of hyperventilation or "deep breathing" through the use of Dr. Buteyko's approach. We teach a child how to eliminate the excessive ventilation of the lungs—that is to say, how to eliminate hyperventilation and to normalize the respiratory function as a whole. Thus, the body no longer has to produce an excessive amount of mucus, which defends against hyperventilation, and the child is given the chance to continuously breathe through the nose. Nasal breathing restores the natural ventilation of the ear, nose and throat area, as well as natural drainage, and the inflammation of the adenoids is halted. In addition to this, the adenoids stop enlarging, or, as is sometimes the case, even get smaller due to the elimination of the mucous membrane and tissue puffiness.

Sasha: *And so, it is my understanding that parents go to an ENT doctor, who measures the adenoids and then on that basis says that surgery is no longer necessary for this child.*

Doctor Novozhilov: Yes. In the majority of cases, Dr. Buteyko's breathing improvement makes it possible to avoid adenoid removal surgery.

Sasha: *And what, on the whole, happens to a child's health when he starts to apply the breathing improvement program?*

Doctor Novozhilov: Dr. Buteyko's method is holistic; that is to say, it restores health in general and does not just eliminate a specific symptom. When the respiratory function is normalized, the child's immune system begins to recover and he stops hurting. His memory and ability to focus improves, and in addition the child becomes calmer. It usually becomes easier for teachers and parents to work with a child and his progress in school improves. Moreover, other problems also dissipate—for example, bed-wetting (nocturnal enuresis), from which many children with adenoids and impaired nasal breathing suffer. Incidentally, parents should pay attention to Dr. Buteyko's approach for treating bed-wetting. If a child had sustained partial hearing loss as a result of ear infection, it then begins to be restored. As previously stated, it often happens that during the first few breathing exercise lessons, a child will say with astonishment, "I can hear again!" This occurs due to the fact that the periods of Buteyko breathing exercises clear up the edema of the ears, nose and throat. I already mentioned it but the effect is so striking that I can speak about it over and over again.

Sasha: *How do children respond to the breathing exercises?*

Doctor Novozhilov: We primarily work with the children in motion and use various physical exercises, which they like very much. The child sees the treatment as a game and develops a trusting relationship with the specialist, which helps achieve the desirable results faster. The alleviation of a child's condition frequently occurs during the first or second lesson and the children think of this as positive experience.

Sasha: *What is the role of the parents?*

Doctor Novozhilov: There will always be parents who are looking for an alternative to surgical intervention and who are willing to fight for a child's health. These parents take part in their child's breathing lessons without question, learn the method, and continue to use it at home. In this instance, success is inevitable! Sometimes, however, we get other parents, who say something like, "I have paid you and in return you must give me back a healthy child. However he becomes healthy does not matter to me—I don't care whether it is through surgery or breathing exercises." These apathetic parents often prove to be an impediment to the healing of their child. Therefore, participation of the parents in learning Dr. Buteyko's method is the key to a child's recovery.

Chapter Four

Testimonials

True stories shared by students at Breathing Center for the benefit of other parents and children:

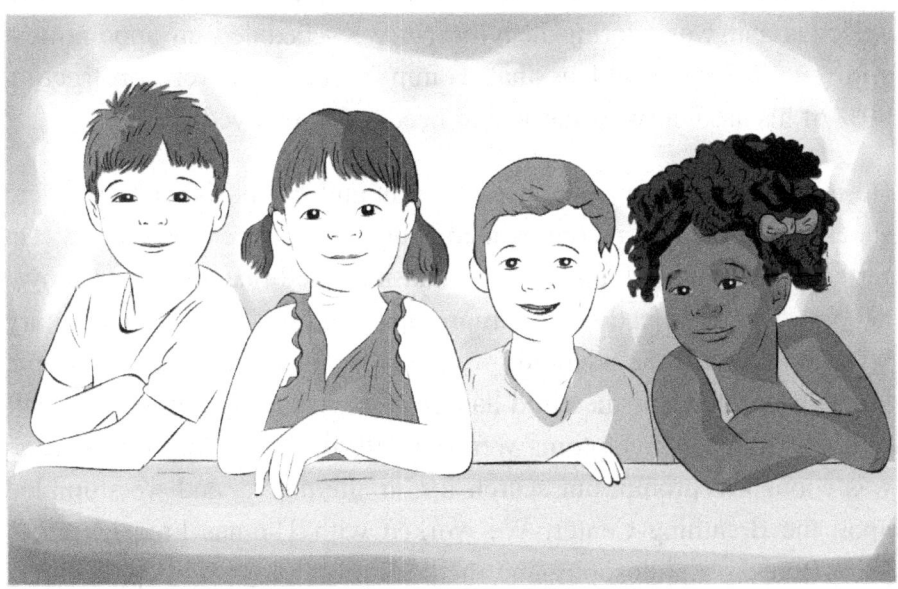

Our 4-year-old son was a mouth breather and drooled often. We got his adenoids removed twice but were worried that they had grown back again, as he started breathing from the mouth again just a few months after his 2nd surgery. Not wanting to get any more surgeries done, we decided to try the Breathing Normalization method and met Lisa Calice through the Breathing Center. Lisa was great with our son and made all the exercises very interesting for him. He looked

forward to his sessions with Ms. Lisa and loved doing his exercises. All the exercises and the recommended dietary changes helped our son tremendously, and he rarely had a cold or stuffy nose again. This helped with reducing his mouth breathing and drooling. We are so grateful to Lisa for her patience and all the help she provided us.
-Tania Tangri

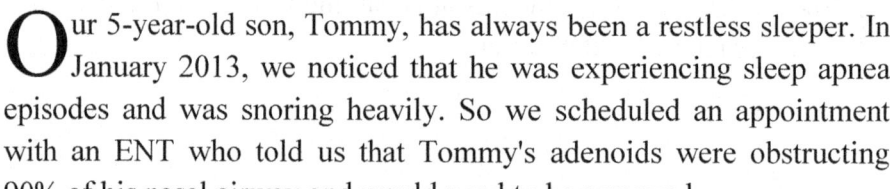

Our 5-year-old son, Tommy, has always been a restless sleeper. In January 2013, we noticed that he was experiencing sleep apnea episodes and was snoring heavily. So we scheduled an appointment with an ENT who told us that Tommy's adenoids were obstructing 90% of his nasal airway and would need to be removed.

He is generally a very healthy little boy and my husband and I were shocked that the first recommended course of treatment be surgery. On further research, we found a study that indicated that adenoid removal is only 25% effective at improving chronic upper respiratory infections. Often, the adenoids would grow back and cause the same kinds of problems as the child had been experiencing before removal! Though Tommy's symptoms were slightly different, that information was enough to prompt our search for an alternative, and we stumbled upon the Breathing Center. We worked with Thomas Fredricksen to learn Buteyko's philosophy and methods of employing his philosophy into our daily lives. Using breathing exercises, modified diet, and general breathing awareness throughout the day has brought relief to Tommy in the form of more peaceful sleep and easier breathing.

Because Tommy loves Star Wars, we encouraged his learning and progress by calling our training his Jedi Knight training. This practice also benefitted the whole family, including mom, dad, and big sister, Ella. We all continue to practice and grow in our healthfulness! Best of all, we feel confident that adenoid removal is no longer necessary. Even if we lose sight of our practice temporarily and symptoms begin to reoccur, we now know what to do to get back on track with our good breathing and good health. - **Joyce Cole**

In September I took my 8-year-old son, Daniel, to an ear, nose and throat doctor because he had been experiencing headaches, frequent earaches, pain in the back of his throat and he was having trouble breathing. He told us that Daniel's adenoids were enlarged and would have to be removed. At first I felt somewhat relieved, because his breathing was gradually getting worse and I was worried he might develop asthma.

His surgery was scheduled for October, and I was hoping that he would be back to good health for his birthday in December. Out of curiosity, I did a web search for alternative adenoids treatments and stumbled upon the *Adenoids without Surgery Program*. So, I called and spoke with a Breathing Normalization specialist who explained to me that enlarged adenoids are the result of chronic hyperventilation (over-breathing). I decided to sign up for *Adenoids Without Surgery* because I learned that adenoids can come back even after surgical removal. The Practitioner described that practicing the Breathing Normalization method will effectively and permanently treat enlarged adenoids without the risk of putting Daniel through multiple surgeries at a young age.

So I postponed Daniel's surgery in order to try the method and see if it would work. We soon started working with Jesse Steinberg in Woodstock, NY. Jesse connected with us right away and explained the theory of Dr. Buteyko's approach; he then led Daniel and me through some breathing exercises. On the ride home from the first session I noticed that Daniel's breathing was not as noisy as usual, and he said that he had fun learning with Jesse.

We continued working with Jesse, and at home I would guide Daniel through the breathing exercises. Sometimes it was difficult to get him motivated, so we had to take a creative approach. Day by day, his symptoms began to disappear! Two weeks later, we saw the ENT again. He was surprised to find that Daniel's nose was now in much better condition (it was now clear with no discharge), as were his ears and throat. His adenoids were still enlarged at that point but surgery had become optional! I was so thankful!

Daniel has since lost all symptoms, is generally calmer and more focused, no longer has headaches, and now has a healthy and quiet breath. And on the last visit to the ENT, he said surgery is no longer recommended! I am so grateful to Jesse and Breathing Center. You have helped my family in a way I didn't think possible!

- Julia Williams

Chapter Five

Breathing and its Measurements

Over-Breathing

According to Dr. Buteyko and Dr. Novozhilov, the cause of adenoid growth is over-breathing. Over-breathing, or hyperventilation, is dangerous for many reasons but primarily because it lowers the CO2 level in the alveoli of the lungs, which, as Dr. Buteyko stated, is the main regulator of most bodily functions. Since hyperventilation can be lethal, the human body will try to protect itself from hyperventilating in various ways, including by enlarging the adenoids.

Reducing air consumption can reduce or eliminate hyperventilation. In a healthy child, the body usually accomplishes this by narrowing the airways through generating excess mucus (leading to a runny or stuffy nose) or coughing. If this tactic is not effective, then the body resorts to stronger defense mechanisms such as gasping for air or enlarging the tonsils and adenoids. By making the adenoids abnormally large, the body is desperately trying to lessen its air exchange.

When a child learns how to breathe less (resulting in increased level of CO^2 in the lungs), hyperventilation is tamed. Then the body no longer needs to come up with compensatory mechanisms, and the symptoms described above are reduced or disappear entirely. Adenoids, for example, are reduced in size down to a point where they no longer bother the child.

It usually takes between two and four months to establish healthy breathing patterns, though the positive results of better breathing become evident within the first two weeks of Breathing Normalization training. The transition from excessive breathing to healthy breathing can be time-consuming, since changing lifelong habits is never easy. But the effort is well worth it: healthy breathing patterns create a solid foundation for optimal health for the rest of the person's life.

Health cannot exist without healthy breathing. When a child's breathing becomes "normal" by Dr. Buteyko's standards (stable Positive Maximum Pause of 60 seconds or higher), he becomes disease-free. That means never having to deal with colds, ear infections, allergies, or any kind of respiratory problems. This is the best gift a parent can offer their child!

Healthy Breathing

Children with enlarged adenoids mainly breathe through their mouth. Their shoulders, chest and stomach often move with every inhalation and exhalation; their breathing is audible and is often followed by wheezing. A child with enlarged adenoids can sit on a sofa watching TV and breathe as heavily as if he is running.

In marked contrast to hyperventilation, healthy breathing is unnoticeable. The ideal breath is so light and gentle that it cannot be observed. It looks as though the person is not breathing at all! His shoulders, chest and stomach barely move, his inhalations and exhalations are silent, and his mouth is closed, unless he is eating or talking.

Nasal breathing is the most important element of healthy breathing. Dr. Buteyko said that any child who breathes through his mouth instead of his nose is seriously ill, regardless of whether or not he expresses disease symptoms.

Through Breathing Normalization training, a child becomes able to breathe through his nose all the time—during studying, socializing, sleeping, talking, eating, and physical activities.

Close Your Mouth

Mouth breathing is often responsible for the flu, as well as many other viral infections. When you breathe through your mouth, you are basically creating a microbe highway from the outside environment directly into your air passages. In addition, the air itself is often over-cooled and unprepared for consumption. A healthy body temperature is 97.88 degrees Fahrenheit. Air any cooler than that contributes to a gradual breakdown of the immune system and can lead to respiratory problems. "Mouth breathing," says Dr. Novozhilov, "is often the sole reason for chronic tonsillitis and enlarged adenoids in children, which causes frequent colds and bronchitis, and eventually ends with surgical intervention."

Nasal breathing is the simple solution, one that you or your child can start practicing right away, and one that Dr. Novozhilov says, "is quite effective in shielding the body against viruses, such as a seasonal flu." A flu virus spreads through infected droplets that fly off a sick person when he coughs, sneezes or even speaks. These droplets can travel up to fifty feet from their source, and are so tiny that they can penetrate even the space between the fibers of a paper or cloth mask. Thus, during a flu pandemic, it is nearly impossible to avoid infected areas and to prevent the virus from finding its way into your body.

Fortunately, the way the virus enters your body can make all the difference. The majority of viruses cannot survive on the mucus membrane of the nose. The microbes in this membrane create a hostile environment for the virus. When breathing through your nose, you are sterilizing the air entering your body, creating a shield against disease. Nasal breathing warms the air, moistens it, and conditions it for perfect consumption.

Healthy nasal breathing is the treatment for enlarged adenoids (and many other health issues) and a way to prevent the problem in the first place. Healthy breathing is simple, although it takes time and energy for any person, adult or child, to unlearn a lifetime's worth of unhealthy breathing habits. Parents need to be patient when teaching their child how to breathe lightly and through the nose only.

While it may be easy for parents to breathe through their noses, it could be extremely arduous for their child if he has enlarged adenoids. This is one of the reasons it is recommended that parents work with a Breathing Normalization specialist who can make this healing journey less difficult.

Sometimes it is almost impossible for a child to breathe through his nose at all, especially at night. In this case, the parent faces a dilemma: should my child breathe through his mouth or should I use medication to open his airways? In this instance, the use of medication is recommended to open the air passages and make it possible for the child to do the breathing exercises. As the child's treatment progresses, medication will not be needed.

It is also important to realize that even though nasal breathing greatly reduces hyperventilation, it does not always stop it. A child who breathes through his nose can still hyperventilate to some degree. The best sign that hyperventilation is eliminated is indicated by greatly improved breathing measurements. (For further information on breathing measurements, see the later section in this chapter.)

Why Does My Child Hyperventilate?

Many parents assume that healthy breathing is supposed to come naturally. They are puzzled about why their child over-breathes.

Healthy or natural breathing is the result of a natural lifestyle. Most modern children don't follow a natural lifestyle, so their breathing patterns are disturbed. Unnatural breathing patterns can be corrected through lifestyle changes in combination with breathing exercises.

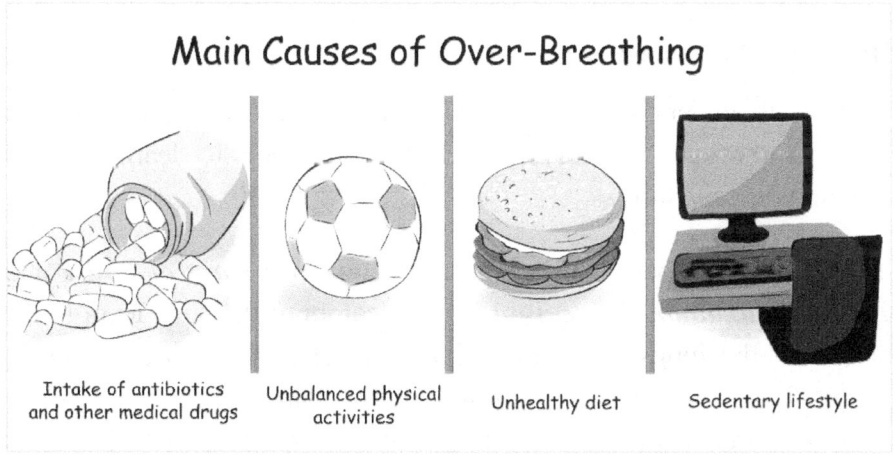

One of the main causes of hyperventilation in children is the intake of antibiotics. Antibiotics do not discriminate; once they enter the body, they not only attack illness-producing bacteria, but also the beneficial bacteria that live in many places throughout the body, most especially in the upper airways and the intestinal tract. When these populations of beneficial bacteria are depleted, the body cannot perform many functions properly, breathing among them.

In the United States, antibiotics are often prescribed to children when they have a common flu, cold or infection. Sometimes, doctors prescribe them as a precaution, worrying that without them a child's ailment might get worse. Considering the harmful effects of antibiotics on breathing and the body in general, doctors at Clinica Buteyko Moscow recommend that parents and doctors practice extreme caution in their application. Antibiotics are useful for life-threatening situations, but it is better to avoid them if a child is only mildly ill. And in every case, healthy breathing is the best protection from any respiratory issues, as well as many other health problems.

Other common causes of hyperventilation include an imbalance of physical activities, improper diet and the stresses of everyday life. These topics are covered in detail in the next chapter as well as other places in this book.

Breathing Measurements

In order to understand the state of your child's health and track his progress through his healing process, you need to learn how to measure his breathing.

There are two types of breathing measurements: **Control Pause** and **Positive Maximum Pause.** Both are indicators of the CO_2 level in the alveoli of the lungs. A certain minimal level of CO_2 in the lungs is essential for good health. A low *Control Pause* or *a low Positive Maximum Pause* shows that the carbon dioxide level in the lungs is insufficient. Higher breathing measurement numbers indicate a higher level of carbon dioxide in the lungs, and therefore, equates with better health. The goal of Breathing Normalization training is to reestablish the normal carbon dioxide level. My experience has shown that some children are not able to achieve this level. However, moving closer to it (to any degree!) proportionally improves the child's state of health. Children who are able to reach a level above normal become extremely healthy—practically disease-free.

For most people the idea of accumulating carbon dioxide seems counterintuitive. We all know that oxygen is essential for life, and we are taught to think of CO_2 as a waste product. Dr. Buteyko pointed out that oxygen cannot be delivered to various organs of the body if the CO_2 level in the lungs is low. Carbon dioxide regulates pH, which regulates oxygen delivery! Unless there is sufficient carbon dioxide in the bloodstream, oxygen molecules "stick" to the red blood cells and cannot be released to the cells that need them. Carbon dioxide is not a nutrient, the way oxygen is; it is more like a key that, when fitted into the chemical lock, releases oxygen. To learn more about this scientific principle, I suggest reading about the *Bohr effect*. Breathing measurements are also indicative of the oxygenation of a child's whole body. As your child's Control Pause rises, you may notice that he will begin to look healthier. The typical pale adenoid look will be replaced with rosy cheeks. He will become more energetic, but also calmer and better able to focus.

How To Take Breathing Measurements

Measuring one's breathing is not a contest to see how long a person can hold his breath! Attempting to hold one's breath as long as possible causes stress, which, in turn, causes hyperventilation. This, of course, is the opposite of what you are trying to achieve.

1. CONTROL PAUSE:

The Control Pause is the length of time a person can comfortably go without taking a breath following a light exhalation. The ability to sense the point at which "comfort" turns into discomfort can take adults weeks of practice to develop. So it's unrealistic to expect a child to be able to do this perfectly. The goal is to sense the moment at which the body wants to inhale. This is quite a subtle sensation, so the best way to approach it is to periodically remind the child of the instructions and ask him if he feels he understands them.

INSTRUCTIONS:

Ask the child to sit in a chair with a hard surface. His mouth has to remain closed throughout the whole measurement. Have him inhale and exhale a few times, paying attention to his breathing. Then, ask him to block his nose <u>after exhaling</u> and stop breathing. When he feels the need to breathe again, he should gently inhale through his nose. This measurement requires very little effort, almost none.

2. POSITIVE MAXIMUM PAUSE:

Description: Positive Maximum Pause is longer than Control Pause and is a bit more difficult to measure. To follow a Positive Maximum Pause measurement a person should still be able to inhale only through his nose, though the inhalation may be slightly forced. With the Positive Maximum Pause, there is always a risk of holding the breath so long that the following inhalation is through the mouth instead of the nose. Avoid this mistake at all costs.

INSTRUCTIONS:

Have the child sit on a chair with a hard surface. His mouth has to remain closed throughout the whole measurement. Ask him to inhale and exhale a few times, paying attention to his breathing. Then, ask him to block his nose <u>after exhalation</u> and pause his breathing. When he feels the need to breathe again, he should *wait a little longer*, and then open his nose and inhale through his nose. This measurement requires a slight effort.

- For very young children, I suggest introducing only the Control Pause. The Positive Maximum Pause may be too confusing for them.

- For older children, I suggest practicing both pauses a few times, so they understand the difference between them. After that, keep it simple by measuring the Control Pause only.

Realistically, when you ask your child to measure his Control Pause, he will be measuring something in between his Control and Positive Maximum pauses. Don't worry—this is to be expected. You need a reference point, which we will call "Control Pause," even if it is a bit higher than an actual Control Pause. A possible range of 2 to 4 seconds is acceptable and not essential at the beginning of a breathing training. What is important is whether the Control Pause increases after doing breathing exercises and over the course of weeks, months and years.

You will need to measure your child's Control Pause (and hopefully your own!) on a daily basis to measure your child's breathing. At the beginning of the training, I suggest measuring the Positive Maximum Pause only occasionally, in order to evaluate your own or your child's state of health more precisely.

Some children are very attached to the idea of achieving a high Control Pause. Of course, attaining high numbers is a good motivator, but it can also lead to cheating. Some children push too hard, inhale slightly through their mouth, or come up with other creative tricks. I remember an eight-year-old boy who tried to please his mother by demonstrating a high Control Pause. According to his breathing measurements, his Control Pause was 7 minutes! Astonishingly, his mother believed him, and even complained to me that, despite his astronomical Control Pause, the boy was still suffering from rhinitis and enlarged adenoids. When I measured his real Control Pause, it was only 12 seconds. Please watch your child's breathing measurements closely!

When To Take Breathing Measurements

- Measure your child's Control Pause first thing every morning. Have him sit, ask him to block his nose and take the measurement. The Morning Control Pause is the most important record of the child's healing journey, so record it every day. You will also need to measure your child's Control Pause before and after each session of breathing exercises.

- For <u>a session without movement</u>, measure the Control Pause before the session and 3 to 5 minutes after the session. I recommend using this brief interlude after the session for relaxation.

- For <u>a session in motion</u>, measure the Control Pause before the session, and then 15, 30, 45 or 60 minutes after it. The number of minutes between the end of the session and when the post-session Control Pause is taken depends on the intensity of the session. If the session was not intense, the post-session Control Pause can be measured after 15 minutes. If it was very intense, wait a full hour before measuring the Control Pause. As a general rule, the post-session Control Pause should be taken once the breathing calms down again, which can take from 15 to 60 minutes after finishing a physical activity.

If you are not sure which length of time to use, try measuring the Control Pause four times—15, 30, 45 and 60 minutes after a session in motion—on successive days, using the same breathing exercise. Use the highest number. This experiment will allow you to determine the best length of time to wait before measuring your post-session Control Pause.

Important: If breathing exercises are done correctly, the post-session Control Pause should be higher than the one before it. A session without movement should generate a Control Pause increase of at least 2 seconds. A session in motion usually generates an increase of at least

5 seconds. If the post-session Control Pause is lower than pre-session one, then the breathing exercises were done incorrectly and produced a negative effect. Always remember to measure both before and after Control Pauses when doing breathing exercises. You will need these measurements to evaluate how effective the application of exercises is.

How To Record Breathing Measurements

Record your child's breathing measurements (as well as your own) in a logbook or journal. The *Breathing Log Book* is an important tool, which you will find in the end of this book. Please use it to keep track of breathing improvement progress.

Here is a sample day:

Tuesday, October 22nd Morning Control Pause—13 seconds.
1st session at 6.30 am: 30 min of seated breath holds. Control Pause before: 15 sec; Control Pause after: 18 seconds.
2nd session at 4 pm: 30 min on a treadmill with breath holds. Control Pause before: 14 seconds; Control Pause after: 19 seconds.
3rd session at 8.30 pm: 30 min (10 min—airplane and other games; in bed—humming, breathing through one nostril and relaxation). Control Pause before: 18 seconds; Control Pause after: 20 seconds.

It is important to track progress over the course of months, both to confirm that what you are doing is actually working and to motivate you to continue the healing process.

How To Read Breathing Measurements

If a child's (or adult's, for that matter) Control Pause is less than 10 seconds, then that person is very ill. For children with enlarged adenoids, this is almost invariably the case, and it should serve as a definite indicator that the child should not be forced to follow the typical hyperactive schedule that most children have today.

Following is a chart created by Dr. Buteyko that shows, in detail, the significance of breathing measurements. Breathing measurements are interpreted in the same way for both children and adults.

The body conditions and criteria of lung ventilation according to Dr. Buteyko:

Health Status	Breathing	Degree Of Abnormality	CO_2 In Alveoli % (Millimeters Of Mercury)		Positive Maximum Pause (Seconds)	Pulse (Beats Per Minute)
Super Endurance Longevity	Gentle Breathing	VII	Special Conditions			
		VI				
		V	7.5	53.5	180	48
		IV	7.4	52.8	150	50
		III	7.3	52	120	52
		II	7.1	50.6	100	55
		I	6.8	48.5	80	57
The Norm (Optimal Health)			6.5	46.3	60	60
Disease	Excessive Breathing	I	6	42.8	50	65
		II	5.5	39.2	40	70
		III	5	35.7	30	75
		IV	4.5	32.1	20	80
		V	4	28.5	10	90
		VII	3.5	25	5	100
DEATH						

The Norm:
According to Dr. Buteyko, a healthy person has a Positive Maximum Pause of 60 seconds, and a Control Pause of more than 30 seconds. This means that for this person, it is easy to go without air for one minute, and extremely easy to do it for half a minute. This person does not have any negative symptoms, and their immune system protects them from seasonal respiratory problems, as well as from many serious health issues. His energy level is high, and his body does not require a great deal of food or sleep in order to rejuvenate. This state of 'perfect health' does not occur when your PMP reaches 60 seconds just once. A person belongs to this category only when his PMP is 60 seconds or higher <u>all the time</u>—day and night—for at least six months.

Today, it is extremely rare to meet someone who belongs to this category. If you do, most likely it would be an athlete or an elderly person living quietly in a rural area.

If your PMP and CP are below the norm, it means that your health is compromised.

1st Level of Hyperventilation:
If your PMP is consistently between 40 and 60 seconds, you are an extremely healthy person. Most likely you don't have any symptoms, and if you do, they don't last long. You have no need for medication, although at this level your immune system is still not strong enough to completely protect you from disease. If you develop a disease, your immune system will be weakened, which will lower your PMP and CP.

2nd Level of Hyperventilation:
If your PMP is in the range of 25 and 40 seconds, you belong to the category of the semi-healthy. You might actually think of yourself as a healthy person, and if so, this means you have health issues you are not aware of or ones you consider normal. For example, you might periodically have headaches, heartburn or constipation. You might

say, *Who doesn't? Isn't it normal?* My answer is, people whose PMP is at the norm don't have these issues. And yes, it is very common, but not normal. These symptoms will go away if you improve your breathing. If your PMP is closer to 25 seconds, you might still have symptoms of various diseases.

3rd Level of Hyperventilation:
If your PMP is between 10 and 25 seconds, you are not healthy. When you breathe in you are breathing in 3 to 6 times more air than your body needs. This creates a very negative impact on all of your body's systems and throws many functions out of balance. You likely have active symptoms and your energy level is low. It is also possible that your mind often feels unclear or you have difficulty concentrating. You are sensitive to weather changes.

4th Level of Hyperventilation:
Dr. Buteyko stated that if someone's PMP is below 10 seconds, he is severely ill, whether they are a child or adult, whether or not they have symptoms, and whether or not they are aware of it. A person from this category is emotionally vulnerable; he may have a poor memory, difficulty focusing, and low self-esteem. This person might experience chronic fatigue or depression, or may get minor injuries. There might be very strong symptoms, and the person might be on strong medication. It is critical for such a person to improve his or her breathing. If they don't, the problem will become increasingly difficult to correct.

5th Level of Hyperventilation:
If a person's PMP is below 5 seconds, he is critically ill—whether he has symptoms or not. This person needs the immediate attention of a Breathing Normalization specialist and a lot of one-on-one work.

The Last Line Of The Chart:
When a person passes away, his CP and PMP becomes zero.

Please note that an intake of steroids and other medical drugs can affect breathing measurements. Steroids always inflate CP and PMP. If you are on steroids, or your child is, keep in mind that the real measurements are significantly lower.

Also, the numbers in the chart above are accurate for locations at sea level. If a person is in a high altitude area, their numbers will be lower. For example, at a higher altitude, a PMP of 40 seconds could be equal to a PMP of 60 seconds, indicating that the person is in optimal health.

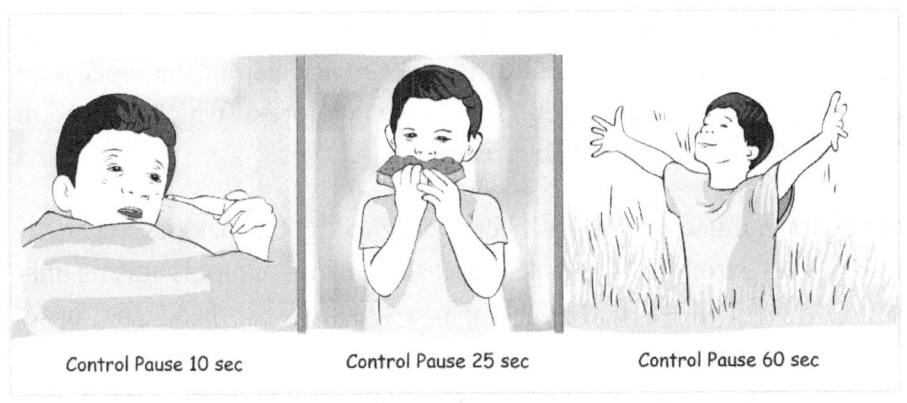

Control Pause 10 sec   Control Pause 25 sec   Control Pause 60 sec

You probably noticed that there is also an upper section in Buteyko's chart. What happens when PMP goes above the norm? Is it even possible? Yes. Many of Dr. Buteyko's students had PMPs of 120 and even 180 seconds, and you, too, can train yourself or your child to get to that level. Many advanced spiritual practitioners, particularly yogis, are at this level. From Dr. Buteyko's perspective, this state of human well-being is extraordinary. When the PMP goes beyond 60 seconds, the person starts to develop certain abilities—for example, his intuition and confidence strengthen, his decision-making process becomes clearer. High PMP also encourages a long and active life.

Please keep in mind the Breathing Normalization method is not a pill and will not change your child's health instantly. I've seen many people become impatient when they do not see instant results. It takes at least six months for the immune, nervous, and other bodily systems to rehabilitate themselves. The training facilitates this process, but there is no way to jump immediately from being an invalid to being superman. Recovery is gradual. Even though this method is the most effective and fastest healing technique I am familiar with, it still requires time.

Healing Crisis

Parents need to be aware of the Healing Crisis as their child recovers from hyperventilation. As the body moves toward balance, there usually comes a point at which symptoms increase or new symptoms appear. This is temporary, and it is a necessary step in the process of restoring health. This is very similar to a process which occurs in homeopathic and other holistic treatments.

Since the immune system has been weakened by the lack of oxygen, as it becomes stronger it attacks disease-causing microorganisms that were dormant in the body. This can result in fever, headache, upset stomach, intestinal upset or other ailments. These are symptoms of the strengthened immune system going after viruses and bacteria and expelling them from the body. They are temporary and are not cause for alarm.

On the path to recovery from hyperventilation, your child will most likely become ill once, twice, or in rare cases, a few times. Most likely the symptoms will appear the same as when your child has a cold or flu. It is very important to let the child go through this process without suppressing the symptoms. It is a sign of the body's successful fight against disease and is required in order to restore health. It is fine to treat the illness with natural remedies if symptoms become bad enough. However, please try your best not to use chemically based medications. If you have to use them, keep it minimal.

During a healing crisis, it is very important for the child to have plenty of rest and to stay warm and comfortable. If possible, keep your child out of school and away from intense physical exertion and over-excitement.

Usually the healing crisis does not last long—just a few days to a week—although in some cases it can extend to two weeks.

A healing crisis often occurs when the Control Pause reaches around 20 seconds. If your child's CP begins stabilizing at around 20 seconds, expect your child to temporarily feel ill, as he will likely go through a healing crisis at that time.

How To Recognize The Healing Crisis

A healing crisis can be confusing—it might look like a virus, suggesting that a child's health is getting worse. To differentiate the healing crisis from a simple disease state, you will need to closely observe your child's breathing measurements. If his Morning Control Pause increases fast (for example, doubling within a couple of weeks), expect a healing crisis. When it starts, the Morning Control Pause will suddenly drop down and the child will not feel good. After the healing crisis is over, his Control Pause will rise again and will stabilize at a new, higher level.

A healing crisis can be scary, and yet it is a very positive event, one that normally brings an improved state of health. Explain this to your child so he can go through his healing crisis without worrying.

Chapter Six

Lifestyle Recommendations

If you are trying to stop your child's hyperventilation, another factor to consider is his lifestyle. Kids often have full schedules from dawn to dusk, leaving little time for play. Yes, many modern children play team sports, but this in itself is a competitive, stressful activity, and nothing like the free form of roaming around outdoors, which was the norm just one generation ago.

On top of this, children often consume too much food; their diet is not healthy, is too rich, and includes too many animal-based foods. They wear too many clothes, often made of synthetic materials; they live in a temperature-controlled environment, breathe polluted air, ride in cars and don't spend enough time outdoors. All these factors combined create an unnatural lifestyle that leads to unnatural breathing patterns.

But what are natural breathing patterns? According to Dr. Buteyko, when a child (or adult) is truly healthy, his breathing automatically pauses for a few seconds after every exhalation, instead of immediately continuing on to the next inhalation. Dr. Buteyko stated that this is the way wild animals breathe. Children in less developed countries whose lifestyle remains more natural often breathe like this. At Breathing Center, we teach parents to alter a child's lifestyle to a more natural healthier direction. As a result, a child develops a natural, automatic halt after exhalation.

Stress Reduction

Traditionally children have had plenty of time to explore, to lie in the grass and look up at the clouds, to curl up in a chair and stare out the window, thinking of nothing or daydreaming, simply allowing their imagination to take them wherever it will.

These activities are relaxing. They serve as an antidote to stress. They are like pressing the reset button so that the system can start afresh.

Many children today have practically every minute of their day scheduled: school, sports, classes after school, homework, etc. And when they do have time to themselves, they often spend it in front of a video screen shooting aliens or hunched over a handheld device texting. Such activities are not relaxing, but rather create more tension and stress.

When a child has time to truly relax, the breathing can settle down, and the body begins to move toward retaining sufficient carbon dioxide. This aspect is explored further in the *Breathing Exercises* section of this book.

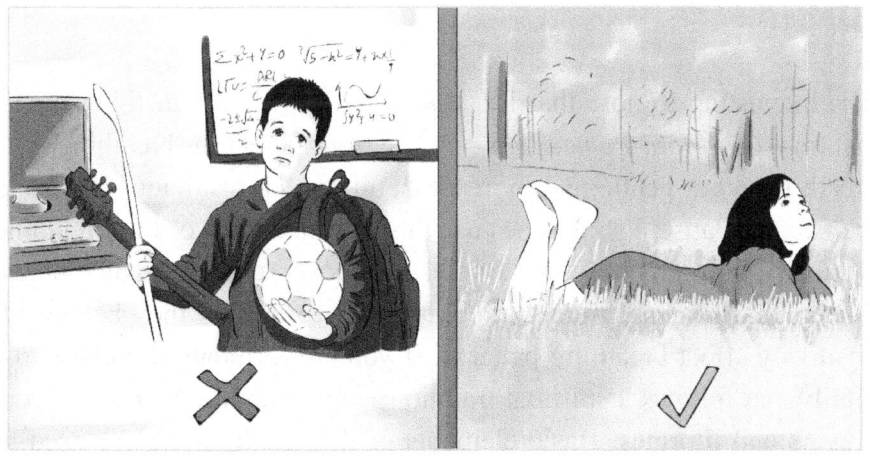

Another essential part of stress reduction is spirituality. Before modern times, many cultures introduced a child to a spiritual tradition as soon as he was born. Among other benefits, this tradition played the very important role of protecting a child from fears and other stresses of daily life. It also acted as a tool for normalizing breathing. At an early age, a child would learn a prayer and develop a personal connection with a spiritual figure—a guardian angel, saint, spiritual teacher, nature spirit, etc. When a child felt insecure, he would immediately start reciting a prayer to call his protector, often accompanied by a visualization.

To illustrate this, I'll tell you a story about Tusha, my daughter. When she was five years old, I took her on a trip to Nepal, where we visited a very long, deep cave. The entrance of the cave was the only opening to the outside. Inside, the only source of light was from small electric bulbs along the walls. When we were nearing the deepest part of the cave, all the light bulbs suddenly turned off. We found ourselves in total darkness and silence. I was scared, worried that we would not be able to make our way back. In contrast, my daughter immediately began reciting a Buddhist mantra—*Om-Mani-Peme-Hum*—which I had taught her a few years back. Because she was able to fully focus on the mantra, she did not get scared. About ten minutes later, the electricity came back on and we were able to walk back out of the cave.

It is interesting to note that Dr. Buteyko discovered that this specific mantra—*Om-Mani-Peme-Hum*—has a strong effect on breathing. The breath becomes gentle and more peaceful, with a resultant increase in the Control Pause. I sometimes use this mantra as part of the Breathing Normalization process. Dr. Buteyko discovered that many ancient prayers and spiritual rituals (no matter what tradition they belong to) positively affect breathing patterns. If you are fortunate to belong to a family that follows a spiritual tradition, don't exclude your child from prayers and liturgies. Basic elements of this tradition can be used as breathing improvement tools.

Breathing During Sleep

Since children are asleep for about one-third of each day, it is critical to address breathing issues during sleep. Nighttime breathing is usually even more excessive than daytime breathing. In addition, since we cannot consciously control over-breathing during sleep, sleeping encourages over-breathing.

Many children with enlarged adenoids sleep with their mouth open. Their respiration is loud and often accompanied by wheezing. They snore and often stop breathing for a while, eventually developing sleep apnea. They often wake up with a stuffy nose or throat and often start coughing right away. All these conditions are caused by over-breathing and can be stopped by light nasal breathing.

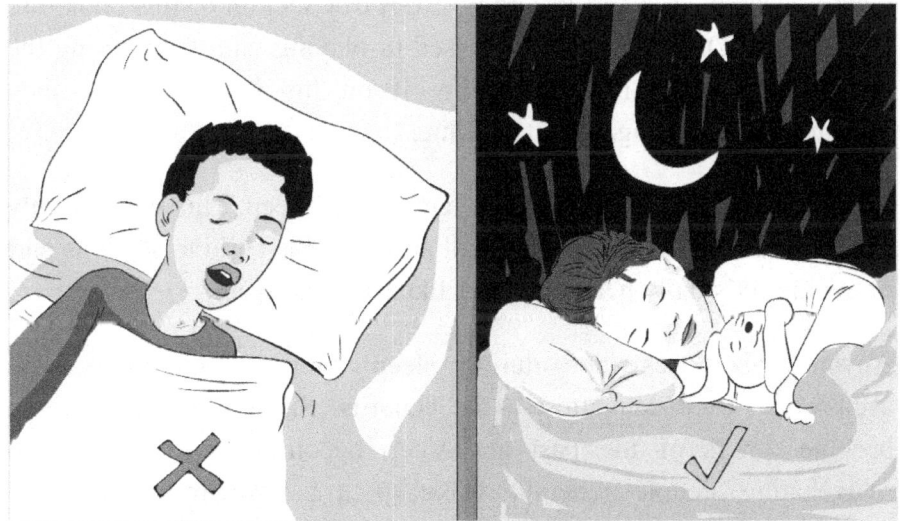

As with daytime practice, the goals of nighttime Breathing Normalization training are:

1. Establishing continuous nasal breathing
2. Reducing air consumption and air exchange.

Tape:
Establishing continuous nasal breathing at night is often achieved by using a gentle paper tape, which is available in most pharmacies. A small piece of this medical tape is placed on a child's lips, vertically, sealing the mouth. The tape acts as a reminder to keep the mouth closed, and encourages breathing through the nose. Although people

often remove the tape in their sleep without realizing it, it provides at least a few hours of support for healthy breathing. Sleeping with the tape on through the whole night normally indicates that a person is capable of breathing exclusively through his nose through the night.

The idea of covering their mouth during sleep can be scary for some children. A good approach to this is to get the child used to wearing tape during the day and, as with so many elements of Breathing Normalization, to make it a family activity. The so-called *Tape Games*, described in the *Breathing Exercises* section of this book, are helpful aids. Once the child gets used to playing with tape during the day and feels comfortable having it on his lips, you can then experiment with using tape at bedtime.

I recommend that parents also use tape during sleep. This will not only benefit your own breathing, but will also help the child to see it as part of the family's daily health routine, like brushing teeth.

Anyone who uses tape during sleep long enough to become accustomed to it can attest to its benefits. Snoring and dry mouth become things of the past and sleep becomes more restful and rejuvenating. People generally wake up in a better mood and with more energy.

Scarf:
Another tool—generally introduced after the child is comfortable with tape—is a lightweight scarf, preferably made of a natural fabric. Its purpose is to reduce air consumption during sleep. This is a useful tool for many children with enlarged adenoids, but especially for those who have sleep apnea.

Wrap the scarf twice around the child's torso, just at the bottom edge of the rib cage, tight enough to keep the breathing in check, but without causing discomfort. Tie it with a knot in the back, so that if you see it come loose during the night, it's easy to re-tie without waking the child. Also, the knot in the back will prevent them from sleeping on their back, which can promote hyperventilation.

The scarf needs to be introduced gradually, first during waking hours, with the participation of the parents and the rest of the family whenever possible.

Other factors:
Many children like to sleep face down—lying on their stomach and often hiding their face in a pillow. This position sometimes frightens parents because of a presumed risk of suffocation. In reality, sleeping on his stomach is the best position for a child's breathing. Breathing is naturally minimized by the child's own weight pressing on the diaphragm, and this helps keep hyperventilation in check. Many children intuitively like this position.

If a child is not comfortable sleeping on his stomach, the next best position for breathing is lying on the side with knees comfortably flexed.

The position to avoid is lying on the back, since this position promotes excessive breathing. In this position, the mouth often falls open, making nasal breathing impossible. When the mouth is open, the airways becomes dehydrated, and the child will often snore, which places more stress on the adenoids and the rest of the throat/nose/ears area. Also, a firm mattress and a firm, tall pillow are conducive to healthy breathing.

Eating a large, heavy meal before going to bed is not recommended. Excessive food, especially eaten late, provokes hyperventilation.

Physical Activity

Children often don't do enough physical activities. They spend many hours sitting in school, in front of the TV or at the computer. To compensate for this sedentary lifestyle, their parents organize various physical activities for them such as aerobics, tennis, soccer, etc. Often, these activities are short, but intense. This is very different from the lifestyle children had in the old days when they were physically active throughout the whole day, helping their parents with various chores and playing outside. The imbalance of physical activities is particularly dangerous for kids who have enlarged adenoids.

It's a common belief that physical activities support health no matter what. But this isn't always true. If a child has a broken ankle, would you say that running is good for him? Of course not! It's the same with breathing—if a child's breathing is weak, strenuous physical activities only worsen his health. The difference between a broken ankle and "broken breathing" is that in the first case the problem is obvious, while in the second it is hidden, since "broken breathing" is not accompanied by bruises and pain. The "wound" remains unseen, and so is usually ignored by parents, who continue to insist that the child play sports without any consideration for how he feels.

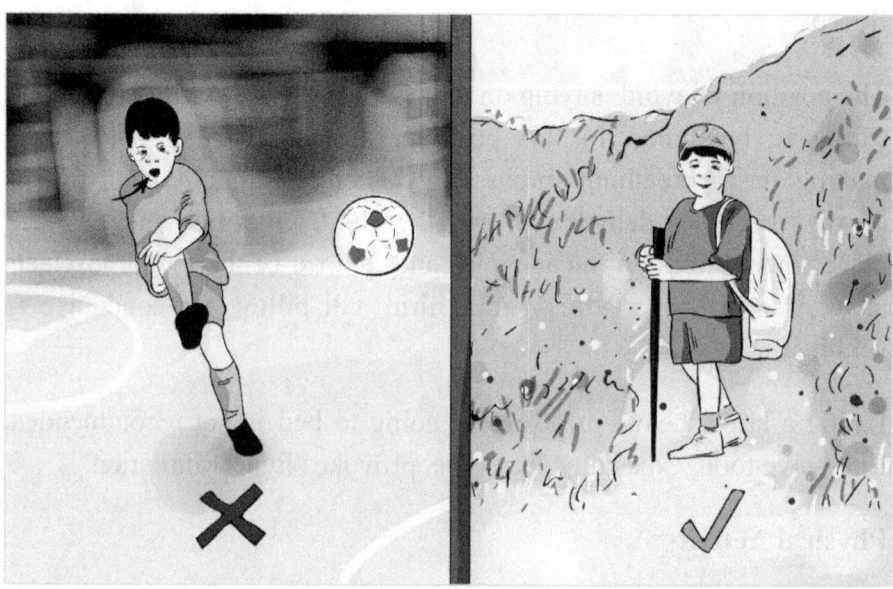

I remember a mother of a four-year old boy with enlarged adenoids whom I met for a Preliminary Consultation. During our conversation, I learned that in addition to enlarged adenoids and frequent colds, her son had only one lung and had been on steroid-based medication since his first year of life. It came as no surprise that this little boy was breathing heavily though his mouth. Nevertheless, he played soccer and swam several times a week. The mother thought her son was lazy because he never wanted to play soccer or swim. But as she proudly shared with me, it was not his choice, and he had to learn how to overcome "his moods." I felt very sorry for this little boy, who may have intuitively known that these physical activities were severely damaging his already weak health.

The first and <u>most important rule of physical activity</u>: It should be accompanied by nasal breathing only. Any physical exercise accompanied by mouth breathing damages the health of a child with enlarged adenoids.

At the beginning of the Breathing Normalization training, I ask parents to observe all their child's physical activities (especially team sports) and to discontinue them if those activities are accompanied by mouth breathing. This halt is only temporary; when their child's breathing becomes stronger, he can once again participate in the same physical activities. By then, those activities become beneficial. Over time, these physical activities (even team sports) can replace breathing exercises and become the main tool for continued breathing and health improvement. However, while the child's breathing is still weak, he needs to do breathing exercises to strengthen it to the point where he can handle workouts while breathing solely through the nose.

Even though parents understand this idea, some are hesitant to implement such a change. The idea that physical activity—sports in particular—is healthy no matter what, is deeply ingrained in American culture. There is also the social element, the worry that their child will be left behind if he does not participate. This pressure can be even more intense for teenagers, since participation in sports can improve their chances of getting into college. Even though a steady routine and the socializing provided by organized sports are important, temporary sacrifices need to be made in order for the child to become healthy.

A child with enlarged adenoids is ill and does not have adequate energy for vigorous physical exercise. They need to be allowed time to rest and to develop healthy breathing patterns, rather than forcing them into activities which are beyond the capacity of their weak respiratory system. This is a short-term measure, and when the child regains his health he will be able to participate fully with the other kids.

Once the child is capable of adequate nasal breathing, he can start participating in physical activities again. At that point, physical activities become important because, according to science, a body in motion actively generates CO_2.

Among all possible physical activities, walking and running are most beneficial for breathing. Until very recently in human history, walking used to be an essential part of everyday life. Children walked to school, adults walked to work, and many people walked or stayed on their feet much of their workday. Now that we have cars and drive practically everywhere—at least in the United States—hardly anyone walks much. This is another contributor to hyperventilation, as walking is a relaxing, mild exercise, which tends to bring breathing back into balance.

Any time you can take a walk with your child, take the opportunity. Walk at a pace that allows your child to breathe comfortably through the nose. If the child begins to breathe heavily, stop right away. Take a break—spend time examining a leaf, or watching squirrels chasing each other around a tree. You will find more information about walking in *Breathing Exercises* section of this book.

Diet

What to drink:
Breathing Normalization suggests drinking plenty of water of the purest quality you can find. It's the only liquid nature created for human consumption, so it best to drink water only. Fresh, seasonal, organic juice is fine, too. Don't let your child drink sodas, caffeinated and vitamin drinks, or low quality bottled juices, since these drinks contain sugar and artificial additives.

What to Eat:
The best diet for children with enlarged adenoids is to eat organic, preferably local and seasonal foods, including plenty of vegetables, fruits, berries, grains, seeds and some nuts.

Dr. Buteyko recommends avoiding animal protein whenever you can. The typical diet with large amounts of animal protein is a serious contributor to hyperventilation. These products cause a reduction in Control Pause and often trigger symptoms. This is especially true for dairy products (particularly cheese), which generate excessive mucus. Various meats and poultry cause similar problems, as does fish, although to a lesser extent.

It is strongly suggested that during the process of Breathing Normalization the intake of all meats and dairy be greatly reduced or stopped completely. At the very least, make sure that your child does not eat animal-based products every day. Once the child significantly increases his Control Pause, the amount of animal products the child consumes can be reevaluated, but it is a key piece of the healing process while taming hyperventilation.

I have seen parents who attributed great importance to breathing exercises and none to their child's diet. They were able to improve their child's health to a certain degree, but not to the level that can be attained if dietary considerations are made.

Junk foods should be cut out completely. Many children crave sweets. At the beginning of the breathing training it is often impossible to eliminate such cravings, but they do decrease when breathing—and metabolism—improves. Until then, try to replace candies containing artificial ingredients with fruits, maple syrup, honey and other naturally sweet products.

I don't recommend allowing children to chew gum. It doesn't benefit them, but it does distract them from maintaining awareness of their breathing.

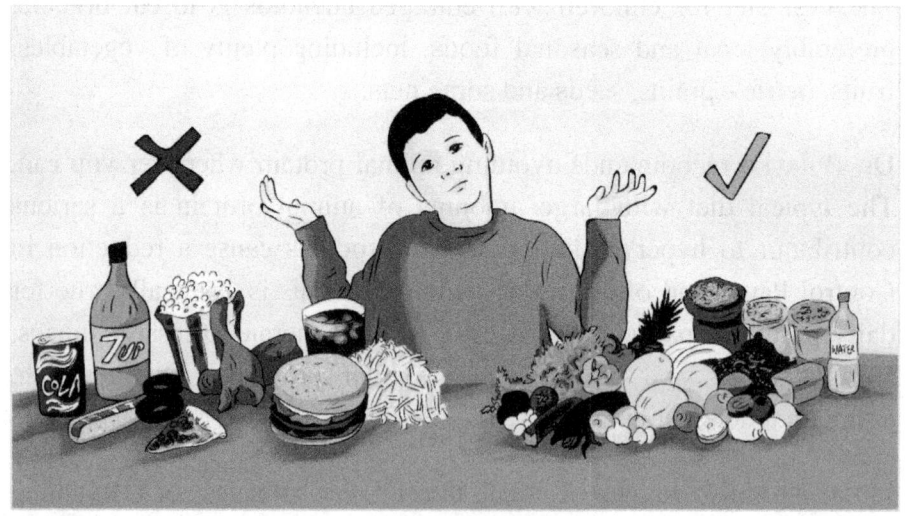

Hunger:
One common misconception among parents is that a child must never feel hungry. Often, parents endlessly offer children snacks, sometimes encouraging them to take seconds at meals and eat more than they want to. Moderate hunger is not harmful; it positively contributes to breathing and health improvement. Conversely, over-eating triggers hyperventilation. Never force a child to eat when he does not feel hungry.

Salt:

Some parents assume that salt should be avoided. For many years, salt had been demonized as a major cause of heart disease and heart attacks. However, recent studies have shown that this is not the case. From Dr. Buteyko's perspective, salt is an essential nutrient and should be part of the daily diet. People who hyperventilate often have mineral deficiencies. These can be restored naturally through salt intake. It is scientifically proven that good salt supports healthy metabolism, improves hydration, helps balance blood sugar and hormones, and is detoxifying.

I recommend using whole, unrefined sea salt—preferably *Himalayan salt* because it is pure and rich in minerals. Commercial table salt, bleached and stripped of minerals, does not, of course, benefit the body. Sea salts are much better, but unfortunately, they are polluted, since the oceans are filled with toxins. Himalayan salt, mined from ancient sea beds, is untainted by modern environmental toxins and provides a rich source of more than 80 trace minerals. Try to cook meals without salt and let members of your family, especially children with enlarged adenoids, add raw salt to their meals according to taste. In the beginning of their breathing training, some children have strong cravings for salt. If your child is one of them, don't worry about it. Let him eat as much salt as he wants. As his breathing improves, his salt consumption will naturally decrease.

Also, some children enjoy holding a salt crystal on their tongue until it dissolves. This can sometimes help reduce respiratory discomfort, especially when it is mucus-related. A glass of warm water with a little bit of Himalayan Salt dissolved in it can also be good for easing respiratory symptoms.

Nature

Spending time in nature is relaxing and healing, and is therefore a powerful antidote to hyperventilation. Fresh air is important for healthy breathing. Make sure that your child spends plenty of time outside.

I also recommend keeping windows open in warm weather. When the weather turns cold, make a habit of opening windows frequently for a short time to let in fresh air. Especially when a child is sick, many parents tend to close all windows and keep the space hot. This is a bad idea—overheating always triggers hyperventilation. Numerous studies have shown that breathing cool, fresh air is most beneficial during active times as well as for rejuvenating sleep.

Excessive clothing also supports hyperventilation since it causes overheating. Children don't like wearing hats, shoes and warm clothes, and parents often need to force the child to get dressed. If circumstances permit, allow your child to wear as few clothes as he wants, especially outside. Being exposed to cool, or even cold air and water, helps build strong immune, nervous and respiratory systems.

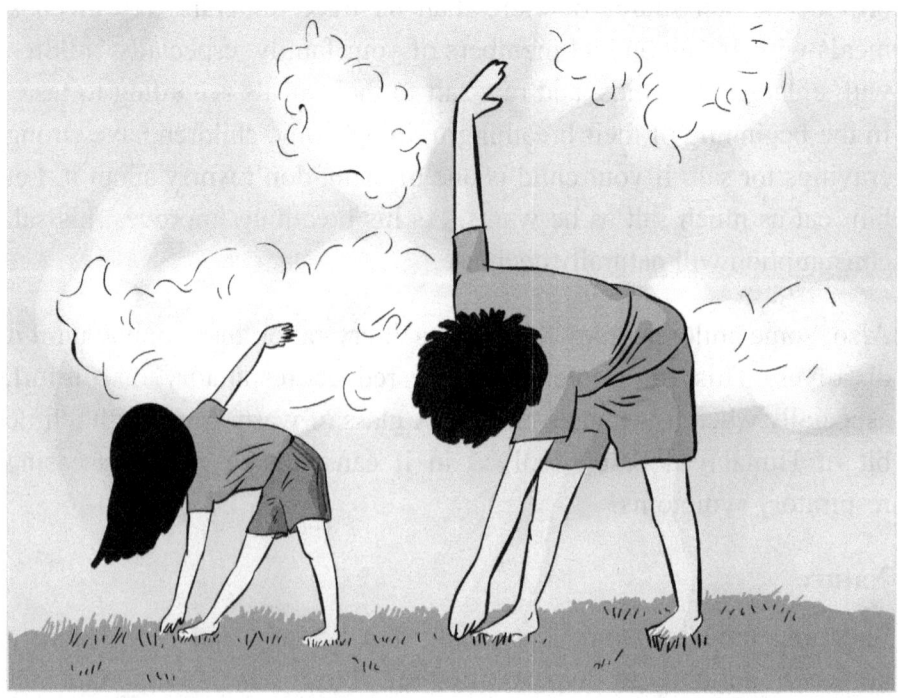

On the other hand, if a child's CP is below 10 to 15 seconds, he needs to be comfortable and warm. Cold temperatures, especially outdoors, can make his condition worse. For children with this condition, wrap a warm scarf around their mouth during cold winter weather to prevent them from breathing in cold air. Do breathing exercises with the child to strengthen his breathing and immune system. When his CP stabilizes above 15 seconds, you can gradually and carefully start exposing him to cold air and water.

The same is true for sunlight, which activates the metabolism and leads to more production of CO_2. Your child needs a lot of it, yet if his level of over-breathing is high, he may have very sensitive skin. He needs to be exposed to sunlight gradually. Be mindful, though, and if your child starts developing signs of sunburn or over-heating, take him inside immediately. Build his strength carefully and gradually, and by the end of summer your child will have a beautiful tan, which is a sign of good breathing and health.

Talking

People don't often realize that when they speak they inhale through their mouth. During Breathing Normalization training, we help people establish complete gentle nasal breathing while they talk. This may sound like a simple task, but it is actually the most challenging part of breathing training. It requires determination and a high level of awareness. Not all children are able to do it. Although nasal breathing while talking is not mandatory for children, it is highly recommended. If you help your child learn to breathe through his nose while talking, he will most likely retain this pattern for the rest of his life. This will protect him from the many health problems associated with mouth breathing, including viruses.

How should you or your child breathe while speaking? Gently inhale through your nose, talk on the exhalation, then pause, inhale through your nose again and continue. While this is simple, it's not easy and often requires months of training. If you'd like to learn how to do breathing exercises specifically for talking, I suggest watching *The Breathing Normalization Method* video training, available on our website on DVD or as a download.

Chapter Seven

Breathing Exercises for Children

These exercises are recommended for children three years and older. With younger children, breathing should be improved primarily by following a lifestyle conducive to healthy breathing. Usually, a Breathing Normalization specialist creates an individual program of breathing exercises tailored to the child's specific situation. For a parent who is not familiar with the breathing improvement work, doing the exercises correctly can be challenging. If you find yourself in this position, I recommend calling the Breathing Center, or emailing us to schedule at least one session with a Breathing Normalization specialist. Most sessions take place over Skype, an online video-calling program. During the session, a specialist will take breathing measurements, select appropriate exercises and personalize them for the child's individual situation. Working with a specialist helps parents create a program that will ensure the child's breathing and health will steadily improve.

Dr. Buteyko emphasized that breathing is very powerful: when done correctly, it strengthens health; when done incorrectly, it quickly impairs health. To avoid mistakes, I recommend parents practice a gentle approach while doing breathing exercises with their child. Keep in mind that if breathing exercises are done improperly, they can impair a child's health. Please exercise mindfulness and caution.

During breathing exercises, a child should keep his lips completely closed and breathe exclusively through his nose. If a child is not able to breathe through his nose, stop the exercise or decrease its intensity. Do the same if you notice increasing signs of hyperventilation, such as noisy breathing, wheezing, or excessive movements of the shoulders, chest or stomach.

- Breathing exercises should not be done on a full stomach. It is always better to do them before a meal.
- Breathing exercises may be done formally in a structured session, or informally throughout the day.

I recommend that a child do three sessions a day—in the morning (before school), in the afternoon (after school) and before dinner or bedtime. Each session takes 30 minutes and often starts with 5 minutes of relaxation, followed by breathing exercises either in a seated position or in motion.

On top of the formal sessions, I recommend doing breathing exercises informally, whenever possible—in the car, on a walk, at recess, in front of the TV, etc. It is important to know how to check the effectiveness of the breathing exercises. There are two indicators: how the child feels and the breathing measurements.

Always carefully observe the child's breathing after a formal session of breathing exercises. Make sure that it has become less pronounced. Ask your child how he is feeling. Also, ask a child to imagine his breathing patterns as ocean waves. You can ask, "Are the waves stormy, wild or peaceful?" If the exercises are done properly, the waves will be peaceful, and the child will always breathe easily and feels better after.

Your observations combined with how your child says he feels provide you with valuable data. However, objective data is needed as well. This can be obtained by taking breathing measurements. To evaluate the results of a formal exercise session, measure your child's Control Pause before and after each session. The pre-session Control Pause is taken in a seated position right before the session. With a session of exercises in motion, the post-session Control Pause should be taken 15 to 30 minutes after the session, once the child's breathing has calmed. If the child was sitting or standing still during the session, the post-session Control Pause should be taken 3 to 5 minutes after the session. In both cases, the child should not eat anything or do anything physically strenuous; otherwise, the post-session Control Pause measurement will be incorrect. The Control Pause after the session should always be higher than the Control Pause before the session. If it is lower, then the exercises were done incorrectly, or perhaps the session was too long, too intense, or not challenging enough. Something will need to be changed in order for the exercises to become effective. The necessary change will vary for each individual and each situation. This is where input from an experienced Breathing Normalization specialist is especially valuable.

Another objective measurement of a child's progress, and perhaps an even more important one, is his Morning Control Pause. A steady increase in the Morning Control Pause indicates that his breathing exercises, both formal and informal, are effective. Since there is no immediate way to check the result of an informal exercise, we can evaluate it only approximately by relying on the Morning Control Pause.

Sometimes, parents aren't sure how to select the right breathing exercises. Normally, a breathing specialist determines the specific exercises that are appropriate for a particular child. I recommend trying all the exercises, or most of them, to determine which ones work best for your child. Pick ones he likes best and those that yield the biggest increase in his Control Pause. Once you have determined the best mix of exercises, let your child practice them for a while. When a child's Control Pause has increased by 5 to 10 seconds, test the exercises again and select new ones if necessary.

A child's breathing improvement greatly depends on the determination, commitment and involvement of his parents or guardians. And even though a parent has to lead the breathing normalization process, to be successful he must also relate to the child as an equal. It never works when a parent tells his child, "You hyperventilate; you are ill; you must do your breathing exercises to get healthy, and I will teach them to you!" The child should not feel like he is ill and weak, while everyone around is just fine. The way to guarantee a child's progress is to set things up as an equal partnership between you and your child from the start. Begin by explaining to your child that correct breathing is essential for health, so the whole family is going to work on improving their breathing together. To work on this, the parents as well as the child (and also possibly his brothers and sisters) are going to do breathing exercises (play breathing games) to help each other.

For parents who have never had breathing difficulties and have never had to struggle to breathe only through the nose, it can be an eye-opening experience to realize how difficult it is to change a mouth breathing habit. Also, don't be surprised if your child's Control Pause soon surpasses your own. It is often easier for children to establish natural breathing patterns than it is for their parents.

One of the pitfalls of parents working with children is that there is sometimes a tendency for them to criticize their child when he breathes incorrectly. Avoid criticism at all costs, because even if the child complies with the correction, being criticized will stress the child, which will increase his hyperventilation and defeat the whole purpose of working on improving the breathing. The most effective way to encourage healthy breathing is through positive reinforcement.

Instead, create circumstances in which the child experiences a sense of success. At the beginning of a first session with a child, I often say to him or her, "I need your help! My memory is not that great and I often forget to breathe through my nose. Any time you notice me breathing through my mouth, please say, 'Sasha, stop breathing through your mouth! It's bad for your health! Remember, breathe through your nose only!'" Throughout the session, I periodically open my mouth and take in air in a deliberately noisy way. The child is always delighted to catch me doing this. I recommend that parents play the same game at home.

Kids love correcting their parents! It's essential that the child experience success. Let your child catch you in a mistake and accept his correction. Without this, the child can feel resentful and put-upon, which can hold up his breathing improvement. So, when your child catches you in a mouth breath, enthusiastically thank him. A positive approach helps children feel good and keeps them eager to continue Breathing Normalization.

It creates a positive context for you to correct your child when you see him breathing through his mouth. What could otherwise be a sensitive moment instead becomes just a part of the breathing game and another success. A light, fun tone is helpful. If you say, "Uh oh, there you go again. Why can't you learn to keep your mouth shut?" you'll get nowhere. Instead say, "Wow! I just saw you breathing through your mouth. I'm glad I'm not the only one who sometimes does that! Good thing I noticed it; now you can switch to healthy nose breathing."

It's crucial for the parent to realize that when a child breathes through the mouth, it's not a failure. It's an opportunity to learn to breathe better. The child has been breathing through his mouth for a while, possibly even his entire life, so, it will take time to develop an entirely new habit.

Don't forget to reward a child for his hard work and achievements. Let's say that for a week, your six-year-old son has had the discipline to do three formal sessions of breathing exercises a day. Acknowledge his success by treating him to his favorite activity. I always recommend that parents give their child a little present when his Control Pause jumps up to the next 5-second range.

I. Breathing Exercises in a Still Position:

I recommend starting Breathing Normalization training by doing this segment of breathing exercises first. Exercises in a motionless position might be slightly boring for an active child, but you can make them more appealing by rewarding the child for his achievements. These still exercises are necessary because they help develop breathing awareness, which is the foundation from which one can modify their breathing. Without this base, doing breathing exercises in motion can be problematic.

Do I Breathe Through my Mouth?

A parent and a child catch each other when one breathes though the mouth. This exercise is described in the first section of this chapter and is repeated below.

This is an informal exercise.

During breathing exercises, a child should keep his lips completely closed and breathe exclusively through his nose. If a child is not able to breathe through his nose, stop the exercise or decrease its intensity. Do the same if you notice increasing signs of hyperventilation, such as noisy breathing, wheezing, or excessive movements of the shoulders, chest or stomach.

- Breathing exercises should not be done on a full stomach. It is always better to do them before a meal.
- Breathing exercises may be done formally in a structured session, or informally throughout the day.

1. American Indian Mother

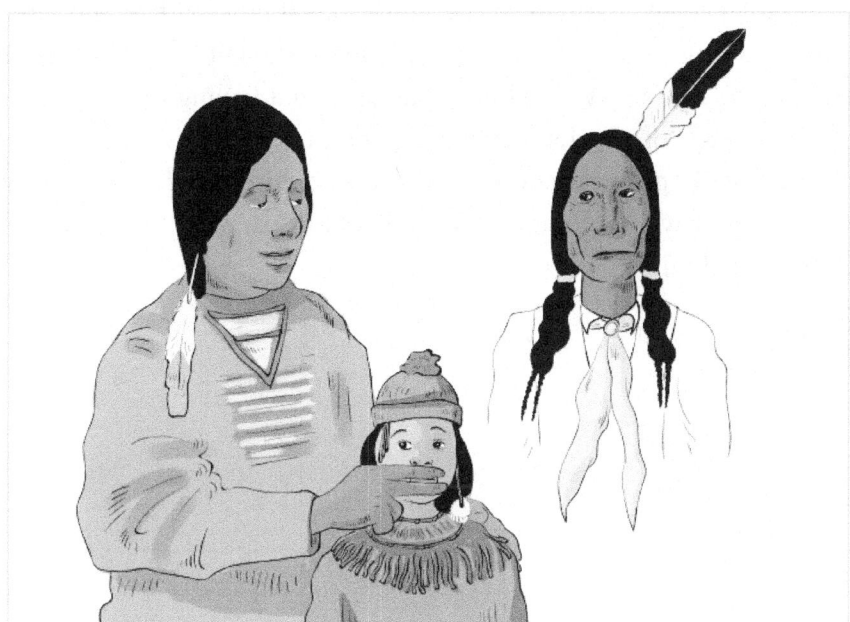

Anthropologists have observed that indigenous peoples who live close to the land and have not been influenced by industrialization know the importance of minimal, nasal breathing. From birth, children are trained to not breathe through the mouth. When a mother sees her child with his mouth open, she gently closes the child's mouth using two fingers. This is done both while children are asleep as well as when they are active.

This is a method that has to be employed carefully and with a lot of awareness on the part of the parent.

A child might feel violated if, out of the blue, their parents start reaching over and closing his mouth at odd moments. This should be done lovingly, mostly as a gentle reminder that the mouth is supposed to remain closed except during eating and talking.

The best approach, again, is to make it into a game and communicate on an equal level. Explain to the child that this is part of the whole family learning to breathe correctly, and that the child should help the parent in the same way. It has to be done with a feeling of joy and fun, not impatience or condemnation. If a child feels stressed, his stress will promote hyperventilation and defeat the purpose of any breathing exercise. Always remember that relaxation is very important for healthy breathing.

This is an informal exercise.

2. Show Me Your Breathing

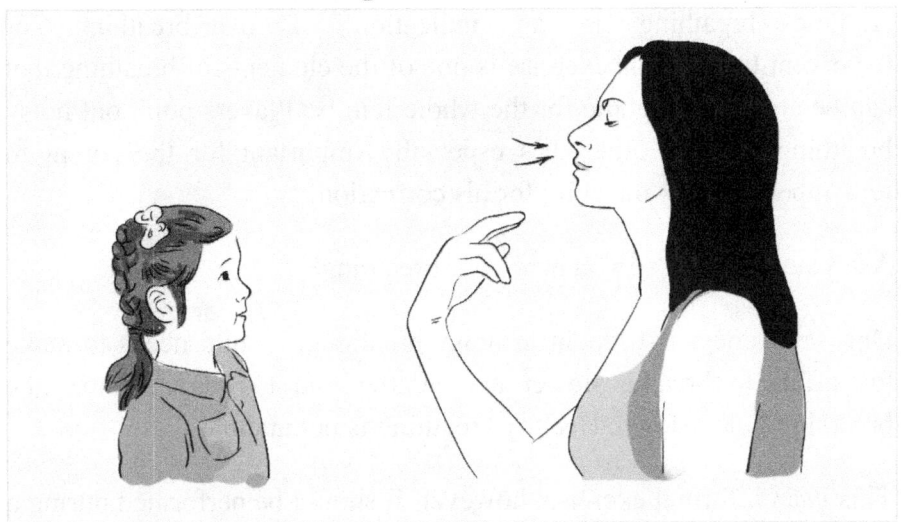

This exercise does not directly contribute to breathing improvement, but for many children it's an essential prerequisite to their breathing training.

Some small children don't realize that they breathe and are unable to distinguish between inhalation and exhalation, so this exercise is designed to make sure that they can.

Use your hand to show inhalation and exhalation, moving it toward and away from your face, to match each inhale and exhale. Then, have the child do the same. If he is confused about it, continue to demonstrate and coach him until he is able to match the movement of his hand with the direction of the breath: inhale, move hand toward the mouth; exhale, move hand away.

This exercise is often done at the beginning of a session. It is also helpful just before a child starts to do breath holds.

Duration: 1 to 3 minutes. This is an informal exercise.

3. Is my Breathing Noisy?

Audible breathing is an indication of over-breathing, or hyperventilation. This exercise is one of the elements of breathing that can be an ongoing game for the whole family. Players point out noisy breathing to each other. It's especially important for the parent to remember to thank the child for his correction.

Ask your child, "Can you hear your breathing?"

Once awareness is brought to noisy breathing, a child needs to make the effort to breathe slower and gentler and to relax, so that the breathing quiets down. Healthy breathing is not audible.

This is an informal exercise; however, it should be performed during a session if the child's breathing suddenly becomes noisy.

4. Are my Shoulders/Chest/Stomach Moving?

Again, a noticeable movement of any part of the body triggered by breathing—while a person is still—is an indicator of hyperventilation.

Ask your child:
- Are your shoulders moving?
- Is your chest moving?
- Is your belly moving?

Once the error is pointed out, a child should practice light breathing with no excessive movement. Parent and child can take turns coaching each other. This is another good opportunity for the parent to deliberately make mistakes, so the child can point them out. It's good if the parent is corrected first, so the child will then feel happier and more comfortable when receiving a correction from the parent.

To do this exercise, the child needs to be still, preferably sitting on a hard chair with a straight back. Make sure the child sits up straight. The child can put one hand on his stomach and another on his chest to check if his shoulders, chest and stomach are moving. At the beginning of Breathing Normalization training, it is impossible for most children—as well as most adults—to stop excessive body movements; however, they can reduce them. Bear in mind that this is a gradual process, and success will come by degrees. The first step is to increase awareness of excessive body movements.

And to reduce such movements? Breathe slower and gentler!

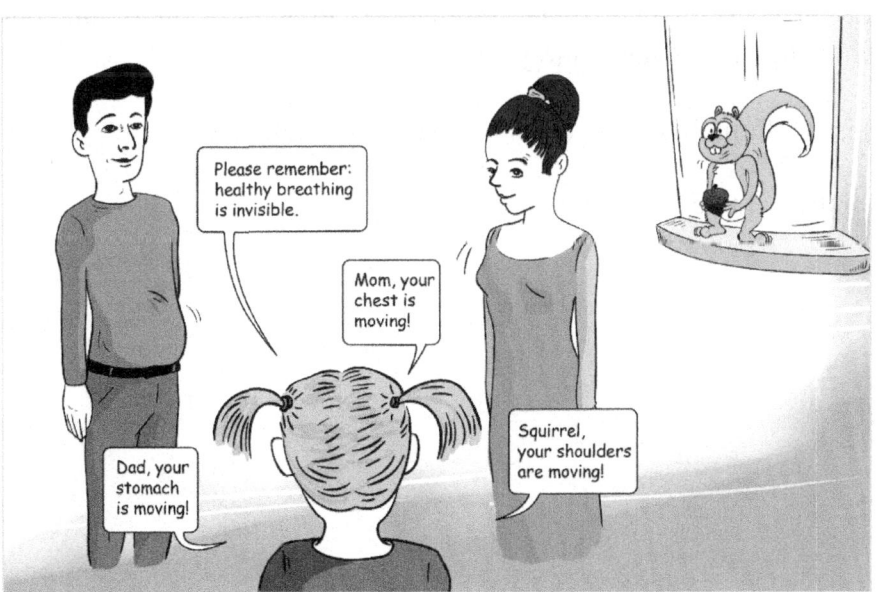

Most of the time this exercise is done during a formal session, but it can also be done informally.

Duration: 5 to 10 minutes.

5. Book on the Belly

Have the child lie on his back with his head supported so it's easy for him to see his belly. Have him place a book on his belly and observe whether it's moving with each breath. The goal is to have the book move as little as possible. This teaches light, gentle, healthy breathing—the opposite of hyperventilation. Remember that healthy breathing is invisible.

Also, ask the child to stop the book from moving for 1 to 2 seconds after an exhalation. If the book stops moving even for one second, acknowledge this as an achievement. It is not easy to stop belly movements from a horizontal position. Try to do this exercise on your own before introducing it to your child.

This is a formal exercise but can be used informally.

Duration: 3 to 5 minutes.

6. Hug a Tree

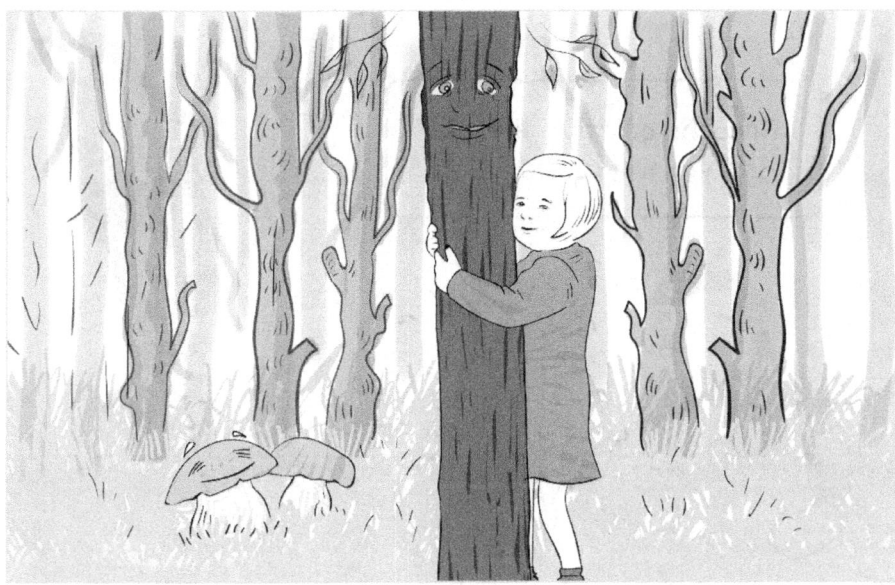

Instead of using a book, use a tree trunk to observe a child's stomach movements. While on a walk, ask the child to hug a tree and gently push his torso into the trunk. Make sure that the child's stomach, chest and shoulders don't move; that his breathing is light and quiet. Remember, a child with enlarged adenoids can only do this when he is relaxed.

Informal exercise.

Duration: 3 to 5 minutes.

7. A Little Mouse

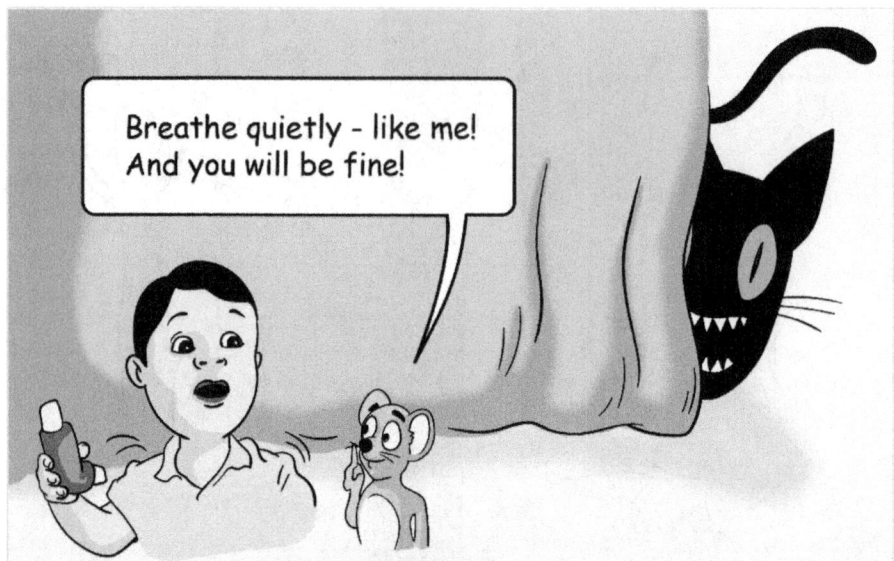

This is one of the best-known Buteyko exercises. Originally, Dr. Buteyko created it for children, but adults, especially those suffering from asthma, have also found it useful.

Tell a child to imagine that Asthma, or any other disease or health issue (for example, Adenoid Removal Surgery) is a giant cat hiding behind a curtain. The cat is watching the child, and if it can see or hear the child breathe, it will pounce and catch him or her. To win, the child must breathe quietly and invisibly (with the mouth closed, shoulders, chest and stomach still) so that the cat won't pounce.

This exercise can be done both formally and informally. It is often used to stop symptoms triggered by hyperventilation.

This is a formal exercise but can be used informally.

Duration: 5 to 10 minutes.

8. Be a Samurai

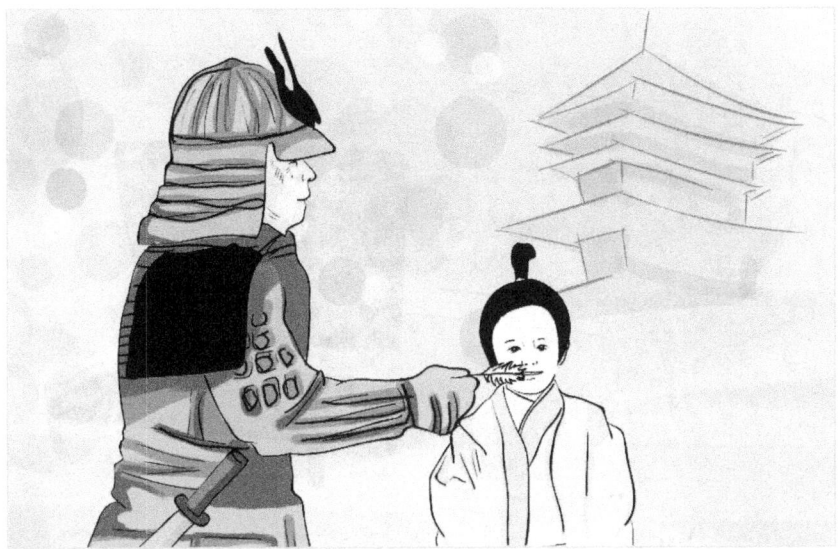

In ancient Japan, a feather was sometimes used to check if an aspiring samurai was breathing gently enough to thereby qualify to be a warrior. The feather was placed under a boy's nose; if he could breathe without moving the feather, he would be accepted. This test might sound strange to most, but it makes total sense to those familiar with Breathing Normalization. Only a person whose health is perfect (on a physical, emotional and psychological level) is capable of breathing without moving the feather.

This same test could be used as a breathing exercise. The game is to hold a feather under the nose and breathe so gently that it moves as little as possible. The advantage of this exercise is that the effects of the breath can be clearly seen.

An alternative is to put a finger under the nose instead of a feather. In this version, the child can feel the flow of his breath instead of seeing it move the feather.

This exercise could be done both during a session and informally.

Duration: 1 to 5 minutes.

9. Tape Exercises

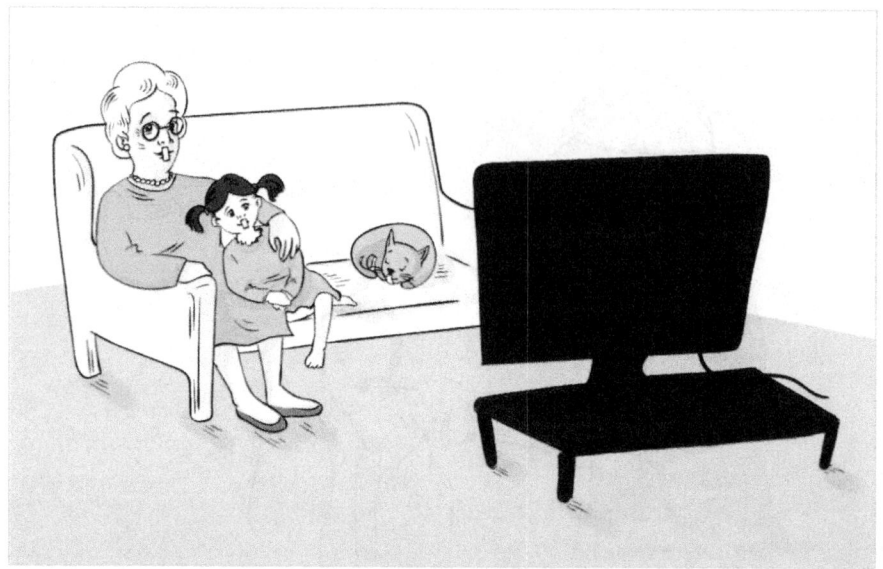

Adults who practice the Breathing Normalization method often sleep with a small piece of medical tape attached across the upper and lower lips. This keeps the mouth closed and prevents snoring, mouth dryness, and most importantly, hyperventilation. At first, this can be challenging or scary. To get children comfortable using the tape at night, start by incorporating it into a game during the day. Aside from preparing a child for using the tape at night, daytime tape games have another purpose: to bring awareness to the lips, which is important in establishing complete nasal breathing.

For these exercises, use only gentle medical paper tape.

A) No Semi-Smile

Many children who hyperventilate almost never close their lips entirely. Often, they keep their lips slightly opened, forming them into what could be called a "semi-smile." You may have seen this look on a child's face and thought, "How cute." It might look cute, but it promotes mouth breathing. To teach a child to keep his lips closed, you will need to use tape.

Another exercise is for the parent and child to wear tape around the house, removing it only when one of you needs to speak. Put a little piece of tape over your mouth, vertically, keeping your lips completely closed. Have the child do the same. Take the tape off any time you need to say something; put it back right after you stop talking. Your child should do the same any time he talks. Many children who hyperventilate are very talkative, and on top of that, they have no awareness of when their speech starts and ends. Because of that, it is difficult for them to put the tape back on when they finish a sentence. This game helps them develop the awareness to close their mouth after they finish speaking.

This is an informal exercise.

B) Who Can Do it Longer?
The parent and the child sit together (perhaps while watching TV), each with a small piece of tape over the mouth. The game is to see who can keep the tape on the longest.

This game teaches a child to keep his lips completely closed for a long period of time. It also allows the child to be silent for an extended period, which is good for breathing.

This is informal exercise.

10. Nose Songs

Nose Songs are a fun way to reduce breathing and counteract hyperventilation. The parent can demonstrate by making up a silly melody, while humming only through the nose. The child can add to it or make up his own song.

Ask the child to create a happy melody, and then make up a sad song—which can be just as silly and fun as the happy song. Try to awaken the child's creativity so the breathing exercises are joyful. Have fun together!

The benefit of this exercise is not only nasal breathing, but also a longer exhalation, which reduces air intake and increases the carbon dioxide level. Why? Because when we are exhaling, we cannot inhale at the same time. A long exhalation reduces the number of inhalations per minute and therefore increases the level of CO_2.

Remember to inhale through the nose only. The mouth should remain closed.

This exercise can be done formally or informally.

Duration: 3 to 7 minutes.

11. Polly's Angel

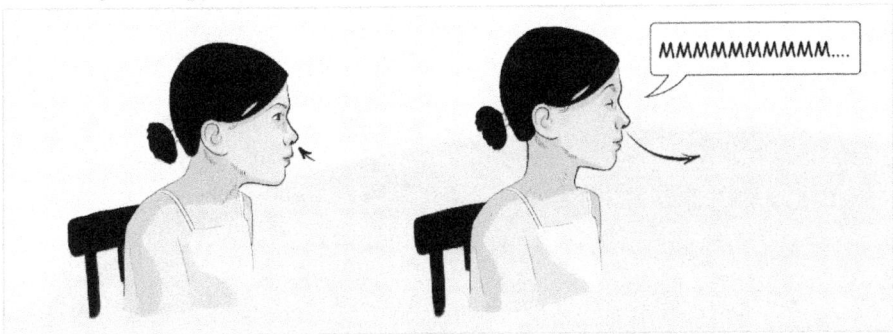

This exercise is named after Polly, a little girl who had severe asthma. She was taking various medications but none that would take away her breathing difficulties. She came up with her own solution by accident. Polly found that when she hummed a long monotone sound, she felt better. Because it was the only thing that made her feel better, she came to the conclusion that it was an Angel making this sound to help her feel better.

Of course, knowing Dr. Buteyko's discovery, we can say that a sustained exhalation curbs hyperventilation and reduces symptoms that act as defense mechanisms against it. For a child with asthma, this effect is usually immediately obvious. Keeping the mouth closed and humming for a long period greatly reduces breathing, so it is helpful to children with enlarged adenoids. This exercise is usually done informally, but can be included in a formal session.

Duration: 3 to 5 minutes.

12. A Sophisticated Device

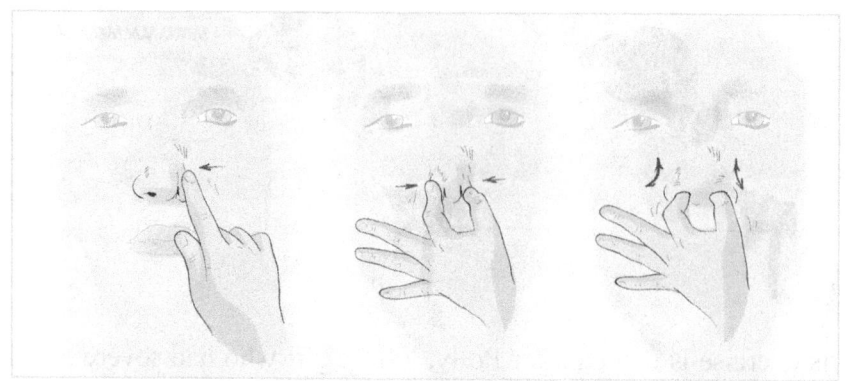

Today's marketplace offers various breathing devices, the purpose of which is to force a person to breathe less by restricting the flow of air. These devices can bring momentary relief. However, they don't change a person's overall condition because they don't foster awareness of mouth and they don't provide breathing modification aids. They often promote mouth breathing. Yet, many people are tempted by breathing devices because they seem like an easy solution. Well, you already have a simple solution. One sophisticated breathing reduction device is always with you: your fingers. By using a finger, you can easily achieve the same effect as that of some well-known breathing devices. There is a variety of ways to do this:

- Block one nostril by pressing on it with a finger or two. Make sure that your breathing does not become forceful or audible and alternate the nostril you block. Congratulations! You just cut your air consumption in half!

- If the exercise above is too difficult, press on both nostrils lightly. Apply a bit of pressure, and then release your fingers to determine the minimum airflow that feels bearable to you. Adjust the pressure so it feels comfortable.

- Another alternative is to use the pad of your finger to partially block the opening of one or both nostrils. You are in control of your airflow—adjust it by moving your finger.

We recommend that parents do these exercises first and then teach their child how to do them. Please keep in mind that for a child with enlarged adenoids this particular exercise might be very difficult! Parents need to be patient and practice a gentle approach.

I recommend starting this as a formal exercise. Once the child is comfortable practicing it, it can be done informally.

Duration: 3 to 5 minutes.

13. Fixed Breath Holds

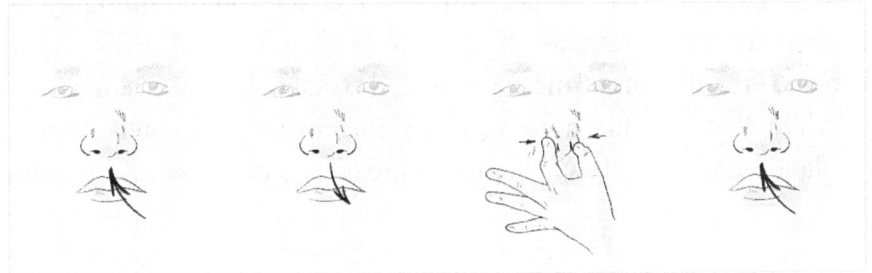

This exercise is practiced in a seated position. Use a hard chair with a hard back. Divide your child's pre-session Control Pause by 3 to determine the number of seconds he can comfortably go without air. For example, if the pre-session Control Pause is 15 seconds, use 5 seconds for the breath holds. Ask your child to block his nose using his fingers for 5 second following an exhale. You will need to count the seconds out loud, so he knows how close he is to the end of a breath hold. This will help him to feel more in control. Once the breath hold is finished, make sure the child gently inhales through his nose. Repeat a breath hold of 5 seconds every minute. Use this minute in between breath holds as a break for the child to breathe normally, calmly, and only through the nose. Breath holds must be done only AFTER exhalation, NOT after inhalation.

This is a formal exercise. Duration: 5 to 30 minutes. Do not exceed 30 minutes.

14. Flexible Breath Holds

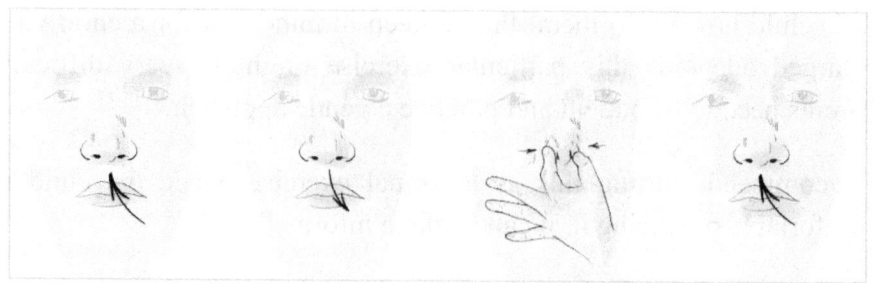

This exercise is the same as a *Fixed Breath Hold, except* that the duration of the breath holds is not fixed. Based on a child's Control Pause, determine the number of seconds he can comfortably go without air. For example, if the pre-session Control Pause is 15 seconds, the duration of the first breath hold should be 5 seconds. Ask the child to block his nose with his fingers for 5 seconds after an exhalation and then slowly start to increase the duration of the breath holds.

For example, the first breath hold is 5 seconds. Repeat it three times, with a minute between each breath holds. Then, ask your child to do a 6-second breath hold. Carefully observe the child's breathing during and after each breath hold. If there are no signs of hyperventilation, continue with the 6-second breath hold for up three times. If there are still no signs of hyperventilation, try 7 seconds; do it three times, then try 8 seconds. If at any moment your child hyperventilates, let him rest until he stops over-breathing, then switch back to shorter breath holds. For example, if the child's breathing becomes loud at the 8-second breath hold, let him rest quietly for 5 minutes, then continue with three 5-second breath holds before starting to build up the time again. Alternately, just switch to *Fixed Breath Holds* and continue doing 5-second breath holds for the remainder of the session. Breath holds should be done only AFTER exhalation, NOT after inhalation.

This is a formal exercise. I recommend doing this exercise for 5 to 30 minutes; do not exceed 30 minutes.

II. Breathing Exercises in Motion

Breathing exercises in motion are more effective than still exercises. However, they can also be dangerous if done incorrectly. Be sure to follow the instructions precisely. The exercises below are listed from the easiest to the most challenging. I recommend starting with the easiest ones.

15. Dancing with a Nose Song

Movement in combination with nasal breathing helps alleviate hyperventilation. When movement and nasal breathing are combined with humming, they become and even more effective tool against hyperventilation. Dance with your child while simultaneously humming nose songs. Have fun! Make sure your child does not move fast; he should inhale only through the nose.

This exercise is mostly used informally; if used formally, I recommend adding it to the beginning or end of a formal session.

Duration: 3 to 10 minutes.

16. Airplane

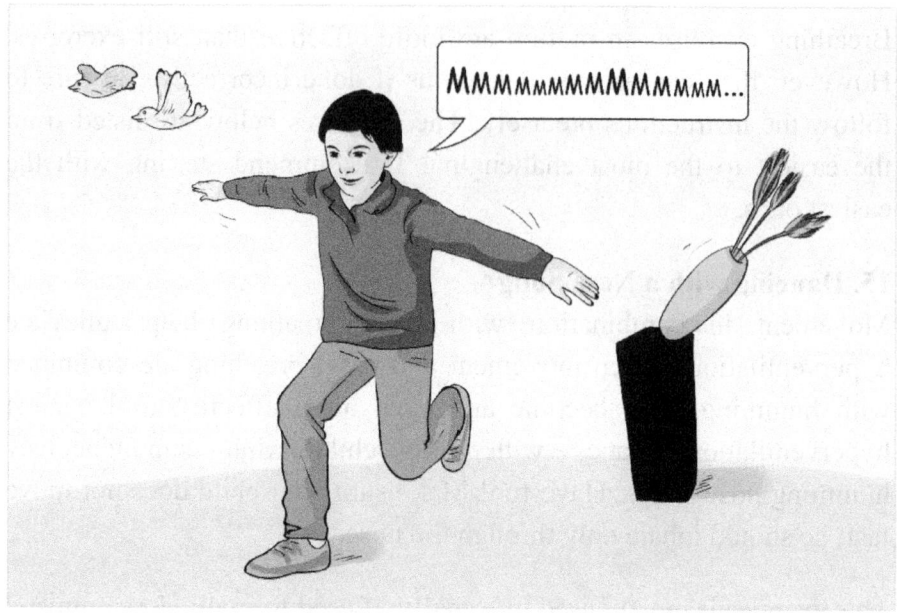

This exercise is a variation on *Polly's Angel*. Ask the child to extend his arms and pretend to fly around the room like an airplane, while imitating the various hums of a plane engine. The mouth should remain closed, with nasal inhalation only. The movements should be slow and gentle.

This exercise is mostly used informally; if used formally, I recommend adding it to the beginning or end of a formal session.

Duration: 3 to 10 minutes.

17. Walking, Hiking, Running

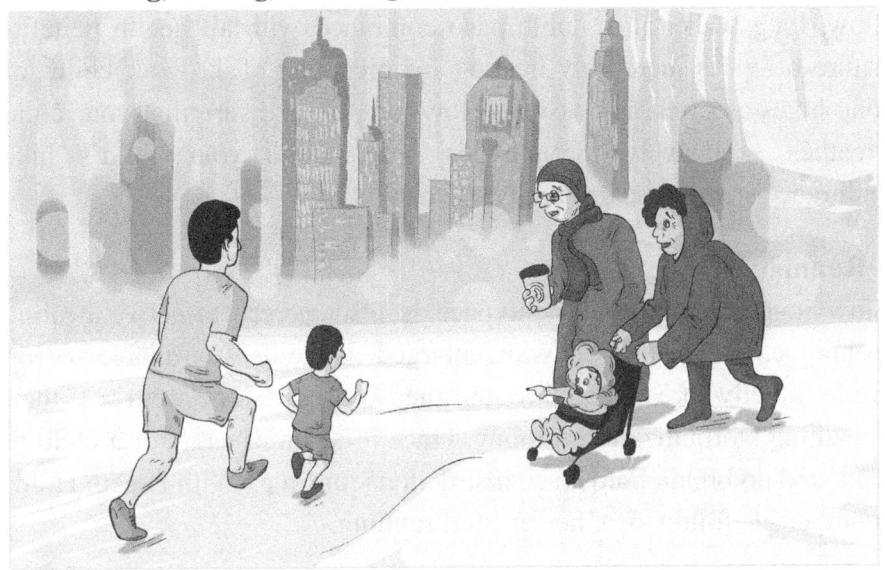

Long walks are one of the best ways to improve breathing and end hyperventilation. Traditionally, long walks were a part of a child's life, but our car-centric culture has changed this. Modern kids are often driven to school, as well as to after-school activities; they don't spend hours playing outside as their parents or grandparents did. The resulting sedentary lifestyle is one of the main causes of hyperventilation. Often, kids are incapable of walking even for thirty minutes. If your child is one of them, you need to start building endurance.

~ Walking
Walk with your child for as long as his breathing allows. The child must breathe through his nose the whole time. This means that he needs to be quiet while walking, or only speak when necessary. If your child's breathing becomes loud or he starts to feel that he needs to open his mouth, slow your walking pace or stop completely to let your child rest. If the child begins gasping, or cannot keep his mouth closed, stop immediately and rest until his breathing returns to normal. If your child's hyperventilation is severe, begin with short walks.

~ Hiking

Slow, long walks at a stable pace combined with all health benefits nature offers is incredibly healing for breathing. Take your child for long hikes as often as possible. How long? Make sure that your child breathes exclusively through his nose. Build your child's hike endurance slowly and gradually. Be patient!

~ Running

Slow jogging at a consistent pace is also a very effective healing technique. Most children with enlarged adenoids aren't able to run while quietly breathing through their noses at the start of their Breathing Normalization training. Once it becomes easy for a child to walk and do breath holds (see instructions for Steps With Breath Holds (number 21, following), he can start running.

Keep in mind that although breathing will become more pronounced and noticeable during running, it needs to remain quiet. If it becomes heavy, stop the exercise or ask your child to walk until his breathing normalizes.

I recommend that parents purchase a treadmill for in-home exercise. This allows a child to practice breathing in motion, regardless of weather conditions, anytime he has an extra 10 or 20 minutes. If a child spends several hours doing his homework, it is important for his health to take walking or running breaks. Make sure that his mouth remains closed. Sometimes, a little piece of tape is helpful in keeping the lips closed.

If a treadmill is not an option, I recommend using a jump rope. The child's mouth should remain closed during jumping. Some parents use a trampoline for the same purposes; however, it is much more difficult to control breathing on a trampoline. Some children end up hyperventilating after jumping on a trampoline—it can be too exciting, making light breathing difficult. These are very effective informal activities.

18. A Corner-to-Corner Walk with Breath Holds

This is a more advanced exercise, or game, and should be given only after the child has reached a consistent Control Pause of 15 seconds.

Ask, "Can you go from one corner of the room to the opposite one without breathing at all?"

If he says yes, ask him to go ahead and do it. Observe carefully to be sure that once breathing resumes, there is no gasp on the inhalation. If there is, go to a smaller room or try an easier exercise!

Breath holds should be done ONLY after exhalation, NOT after inhalation.

This exercise may be used formally or informally.

Duration: I recommend doing this exercise for 5 to 10 minutes. Make sure the child has about a 2 minute between breath holds to breathe normally and relax.

19. Don't Miss the Fridge

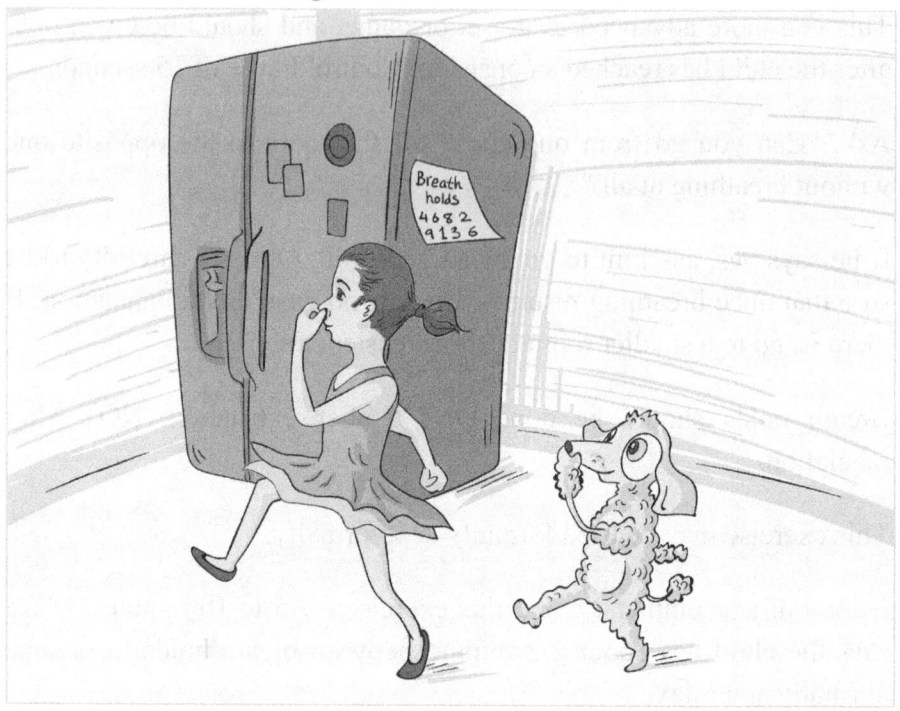

Designate a large object somewhere in the house, say a fridge or a table, and ask your child to do a breath hold every time he passes by the object. The breath hold can be two or three seconds, nothing extreme. This keeps bringing attention back to the breath and balances it by limiting breathing for a few moments.

You will need to participate in this exercise too, so that it feels like a fun game for your child. You can even keep score! Delight your child by letting him catch you occasionally forgetting to do a breath hold when you walk by the fridge.

This exercise should be done periodically; it is used only informally.

20. Steps with Breath Holds

Sometimes, I meet children who learned this particular Buteyko™ exercise from someone who is not authorized to teach Buteyko™ Breathing Normalization. The results are often negative and make the child feel worse. That's because instructions from unauthorized sources often suggest combining steps with a maximum length of breath holds. This actually strengthens hyperventilation and discourages healthy breathing!

Ask your child to walk around. He should start by taking soft steps; if his breathing allows, later in the exercise he can make his steps more pronounced by lifting his legs higher and stepping down forcefully.

Next, ask your child to do a breath hold while walking. The breath hold should be easy—around 2 seconds. When the breath hold is finished, the child should continue walking in the manner described above for about 2 minutes. Then, repeat the same length breath hold. If the child does not display signs of hyperventilation, start increasing the length of the breath holds by 1 second at a time, and continue doing breath holds every 2 minutes. Never ask your child to do a maximum breath hold. Breathing Normalization requires a gentle approach. Straining only produces negative results.

Breath holds should be done ONLY after exhalation, NOT after inhalation.

This is an excellent exercise to use during a formal session.

Duration: 5 to 30 minutes. Do not exceed 30 minutes.

21. Walk with Breath Holds

Walking to school or to the bus stop is a perfect opportunity for breathing exercises. While walking, the child holds his breath for just a few seconds. He then breathes normally, through the nose, for 2 minutes or a bit longer. He then repeats this many times over.

If you can determine the pace at which your child normally walks to the bus, you can then translate the duration of a breath hold and a 2–minute break in between into an appropriate number of steps. This is an easy way for the child to keep track of his progress without having to rely on a clock. For example, a child can do a breath hold for 5 steps, then breathe normally for 160 steps, then take 5 steps without breathing again, and then repeat the cycle.

Breath holds should be slightly challenging, and yet should not cause any signs of hyperventilation. If they do, they are too long and should be modified right away.

Remember that breath holds should be done ONLY after exhalation, NOT after inhalation.

I recommend doing this exercise for 5 to 30 minutes. Do not exceed 30 minutes.

22. Simple Jumps

Have the child do a breath hold after an exhalation by blocking his nose with his fingers. Then, with the breath held, ask him to jump energetically once or a few times. Make sure the child's mouth is closed while jumping. Afterwards, he should resume normal nasal breathing.

Next, have the child walk around a room or dance slowly for two minutes, continuing to breathe normally and calmly.

Then repeat the same number of jumps, followed by more walking.

This exercise could be done periodically throughout the day. It can come in handy if, for example, Mom is making dinner and can't fully engage with the child. She can just ask him do a few jumps, and supervise minimally, making sure the child doesn't show signs of hyperventilation.

These exercises could be done informally or as a part of a formal session.

Duration: 5 to 15 minutes.

23. Three-Fold Jumps

This is one of the most important exercises for kids. It can be used as a primary breathing improvement exercise.

There are three parts to each set: jumping, running in place, and walking.

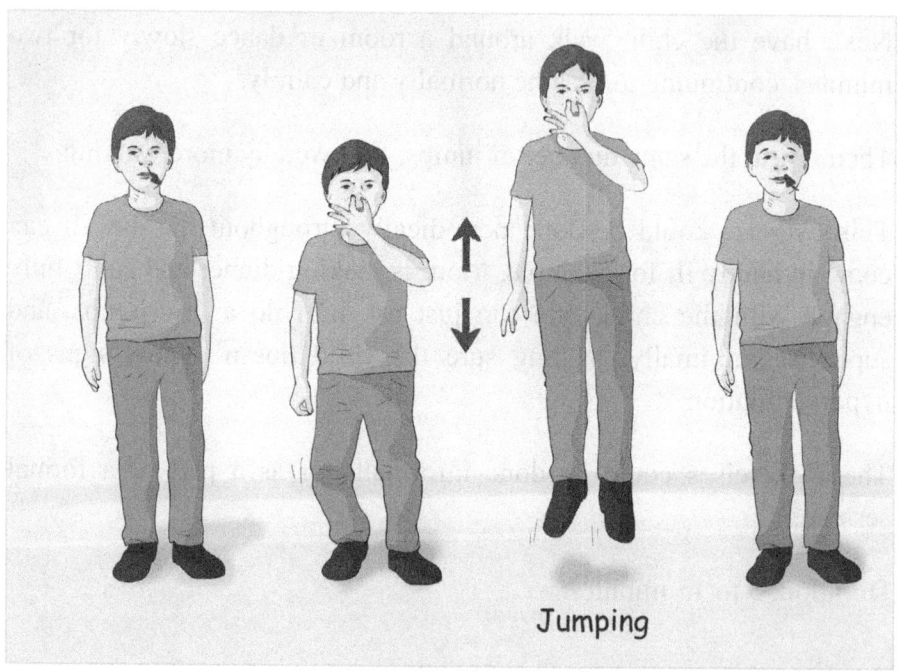

Jumping

~ Jumping:

Have the child do a breath hold by blocking his nose with his fingers after an exhalation and then, with the breath still held, have him jump as many times as he can. (Start with one jump when first introducing this exercise or when a child's Control Pause is very low.) Make sure the child's mouth remains closed throughout.

This exercise should not trigger any signs of hyperventilation. If it does, reduce the number of jumps. The duration is determined by the number of jumps a child is capable of doing.

~ Running:

Following the last jump in a series, the child should release his nose and inhale through the nose. This first inhalation can sometimes be forceful and loud. To avoid this, explain how to divide one long inhalation into a series of smaller ones—inhaling rapidly, with several short pauses and without exhaling, similar to a dog sniffing. As soon as the child resumes breathing, he should start running as intensely as he can. He can run in place. If this exercise is done outside, don't let the child leave your sight because you will need to observe his breathing, especially at the beginning. As always, make sure he's not breathing through his mouth.

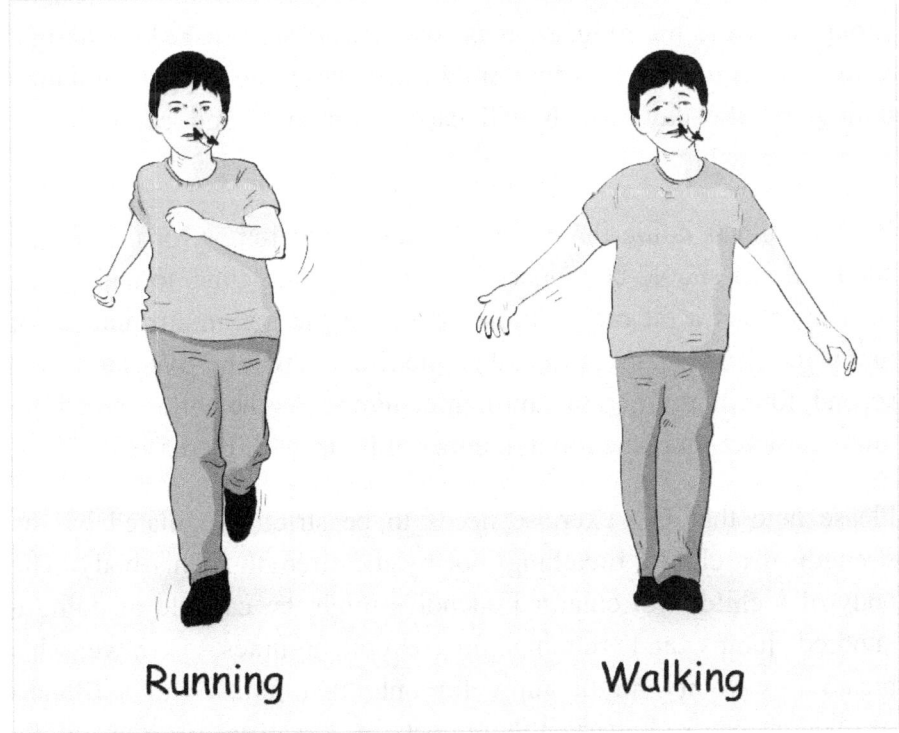

~ Walking:

Next, ask your child to walk around the room calmly or dance around slowly. This time is used to give the breathing a break from the stress of the two previous phases. During this phase, the child should breathe through his nose, but without attempting to modify his breathing.

Make sure the child doesn't talk during the walking section.

This last phase should last about 5 minutes. However, if a child is breathing heavily, he should walk calmly until his breathing quiets down.

This three-fold set can be done as a complete exercise. For best results, I recommend doing three sets of this exercise in a row every day, one to three times a day. It is great for the child to do this three-fold exercise every morning before breakfast. Hyperventilation is usually strongest in the morning, so it is essential to stop or reduce it right away. If you don't, your child will continue hyperventilating throughout the day, which will cause symptoms and contribute to adenoid growth.

If your child is doing three sets, the number of jumps for the second and third sets should be reduced by one jump each time, to make each subsequent set a bit easier. For example, if the maximum number of jumps the child can do is five, then the first set will be five jumps, the second, four jumps, and the third, three jumps. As the child's breathing improves over time, the initial number of jumps will increase.

Please note that this exercise needs to be strictly regulated by the strength of a child's breathing, not by the strength of his body. The body of a child with enlarged adenoids might be capable of doing a hundred jumps and running for several minutes. However, his breathing capacity might allow for only two jumps and a fifteen-second run before hyperventilation sets in. Be aware of your child's breathing, and teach him to be mindful of his limitations! If these limitations are ignored, this exercise will have a negative effect, and enlarged adenoids will only get worse.

Keep in mind that this is a powerful exercise and should be treated with caution.

Duration: 5 to 20 minutes.

This is one of the most important and most effective exercises for kids. It can be used as a main breathing improvement exercise. This exercise is always used as a part of a formal session at first, but can be used informally once a child learns how to do it during his formal sessions.

III. Breathing Exercises for Relaxation

Hyperventilation is reduced when a person is relaxed. Therefore, relaxation is an effective way to tame over-breathing.

Unfortunately, most kids have little space in their lives to relax. Their daily schedules are often filled with one activity after another: school, chorus, hockey, birthday parties, dance lessons, math tutoring, etc. It can become close to a full-time job for a parent to coordinate all these activities. The old days when children used to spend hours daydreaming or creating fantasy worlds with their friends are over for many kids today. The achievement-oriented lifestyle, often imposed on a child from a very young age, creates enormous stress and triggers over-breathing.

To maintain mental balance, kids should be allowed to spend time in their inner world. Being in an interior space counterbalances the stresses of the outside world and fosters calmness. We need to create opportunities for children to spend time in their inner world because it aids healthy breathing and overall health.

I recommend starting a session of formal breathing exercises with 5 to 10 minutes of relaxation. You don't need to relax before every session, but do it often.

24. Imagine

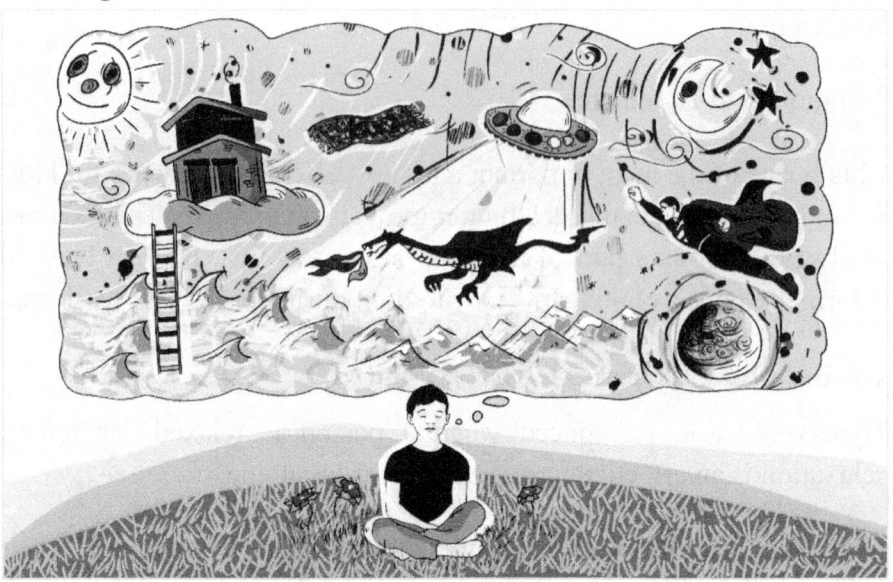

Have your child close his eyes and gently roll them upward as if he's watching a movie on a screen above his head (having the eyes in this position reduces breathing). Ask him to imagine something he really likes on the screen, such as his favorite animal, brother or sister, best friend, favorite car, or a beautiful princess. Have him look at every detail of the image.

For example, ask:

"Can you see the dog's tail? Is it long or short? Is it wagging? What color is it?"

"Can you see the dog's eyes? Are they closed or open? What color are the dog's eyes? Are they happy or sad?"

After helping your child establish a mental image, start imagining with him. Ask your child to imagine the dog flying through the sky, having a great time racing around the clouds, over rainbows, etc. Have the child picture himself in the sky with his dog, flying together and meeting all kinds of imaginary beings. Suggest that he listen to the clouds and rainbows talking to him or his dog. The point is that the child exercises his imagination, experiences the freedom and joy of the inner world where the stresses of the outside world do not exist. Enjoy this mental vacation together!

This exercise is always beneficial, but especially so when the child is a bit tired, like right before bedtime. This is a fun exercise and cannot be overdone.

25. I am Not a Robot
In today's world, there is a lot of structure and restriction in kids' lives. There is less time for free play outdoors than there was a generation ago, and it is now considered normal for kids to spend hours in one position, barely moving at all while doing their homework, or for them to have their eyes locked on a computer screen. Even when children are physically active, their movements are often dictated by instructions from their coach, dance teacher, teammates, etc. If you analyze all the movements a child goes through each day, most likely you will find that it is a chain of repeated, organized "robot-like" movements devoid of improvisation and spontaneity.

The purpose of this exercise is to allow a child to move in spontaneous funny, offbeat and unpredictable ways. A child was asked to imagine a drunken person who makes all kinds of erratic and perhaps comical movements. Next, they were asked to impersonate a drunken person. Children love this exercise but—no surprise—parents would often find it "socially unacceptable." To be diplomatic, I renamed this exercise "I am not a Robot!" The essence of this relaxation exercise remains the same: to let a child's body choose how it wants to move for once, instead of following his mind, an adult's guidelines, or social norms.

Duration: 5 to 10 minutes. This is a great informal exercise. It can also be done at the beginning of a formal session to help the child relax.

26. Heating Pad

Hyperventilation can also be reduced by physically relaxing the muscles, especially muscles in the chest. A heating pad can help relax chest muscles. When your child is watching TV or involved in any other quiet activity, offer him a warm heating pad or hot water bottle to put on his chest or the area in between the two sides of the rib cage, which is where the diaphragm is (the most important muscle for breathing). Watch to see if the signs of hyperventilation—such as heavy or loud breathing or wheezing—subside.

Sometimes, the same effect can be achieved by taking a hot shower or sitting in front of a heater or a fire. The bright orange colors of a fire create an additional positive color-therapy effect for children suffering from over-breathing.

Duration: 15 minutes or more.

This should be done informally.

27. Tense Up

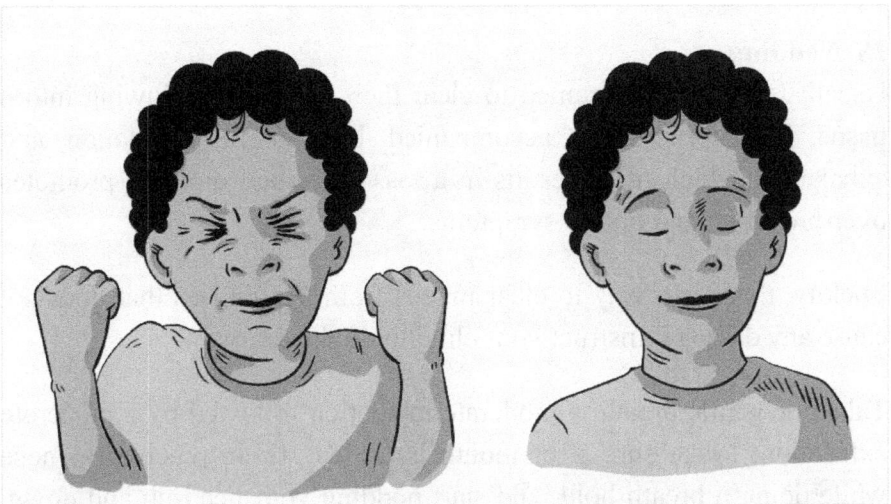

This exercise helps relax the upper body and increase a child's understanding about sensations created through relaxation.

Ask your child to make his face as tense as possible, so that it is a tight, wrinkled cringe. Have him hold this expression for a few seconds, and then have him relax his face. *Repeat three times.* Have him do the same thing in the throat and shoulders. *Repeat three times.* Have him do the same thing in the chest area. *Repeat three times.*

At the end of the exercise, ask your child how the different areas of his body felt when he relaxed them. Give him plenty of time to analyze and express his feelings. Make sure he understands the difference between tension and relaxation. In the future, if you want your child to relax, you can use his memory of this exercise as a reference point.

Duration: 5 to 10 minutes.

This is a great informal exercise, which can also be done at the beginning of a formal session to help the child relax.

IV. Breathing Exercises to Stop Symptoms

28. Nodding

Usually, children are trained to clear their sinuses by blowing into a tissue. This process is accompanied by forceful inhalation and exhalation, which often results in a loss of carbon dioxide, promotes over-breathing and boosts symptoms.

Luckily, there is a way to clear mucus from the sinuses that does not cause any damage. Instruct your child to do the following:

Take one gentle breath: a moderate inhalation followed by a moderate exhalation. Make sure your mouth is closed. Then, pinch your nose while doing a breath hold, and start nodding your head up and down. Do it one, two or three times. Rest a little and then repeat.

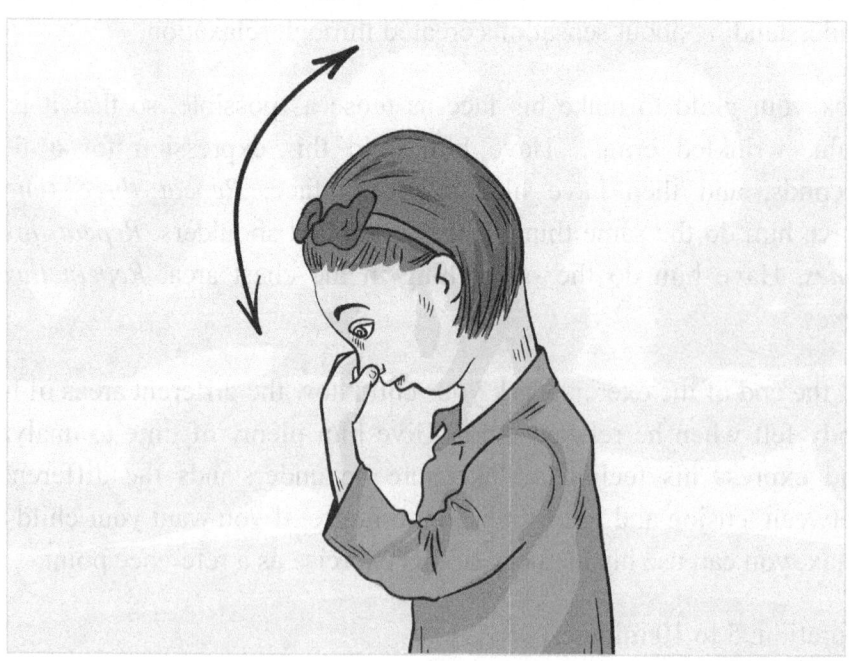

This exercise is often more successful, and more of a game, if the child jumps up and down, synchronizing jumps with the nodding of her head.

29. The Breathing Guru

This exercise is not easy. It requires awareness and patience and not every child (or even adult) is able to do it!

Sit quietly and allow the body and the mind to rest. Make sure your mouth is closed and bring your awareness to the passage of air through your nose. Notice how much air your nose is allowing to pass through without any effort on your part. Relax into slow, gentle breathing.

The body is intelligent and knows exactly how much air it needs. The mind is in the habit of overriding it. If you breathe exactly as much air as your nose allows, you will significantly reduce your air intake, reducing hyperventilation. The symptoms (stuffy or runny nose, which arises as a defense mechanism against over-breathing) will decrease.

If this exercise is done correctly, it is very effective. It will stop a runny nose within about 10 minutes.

The nose is probably the most underappreciated organ in the entire body. Yet, it is one of the most important ones, since its function is to condition air for our consumption and to regulate our air intake. This process determines the level of CO_2 in our lungs, which Dr. Buteyko called the main regulator for all functions of the body. Our health greatly depends on the nose. I call the nose "The Breathing Guru." There is no Breathing Normalization expert who can determine precisely how much air you need at each specific moment, but your nose can! While doing this exercise, take time to acknowledge the important role of this organ. You may want to say "thank you" to your nose to compensate for all the times you were irritated by your nose's attempts to protect your body from hyperventilation. Please explain the nose's importance and function to your child. When a child understands the function of his nose, he becomes much more successful in normalizing his breathing.

30. Coughing

Coughing is another activity that can easily result in a loss of carbon dioxide, thus promoting hyperventilation and strengthening symptoms. Typically, we cough to expel mucus from the throat, which may be necessary, but can be done in a way that doesn't cause problems.

Make sure your mouth is closed, making a gentle coughing sound three times. After that, pinch your nostrils and do a breath hold for 1 to 3 seconds. Finally, open your nose and inhale through it in a measured way.

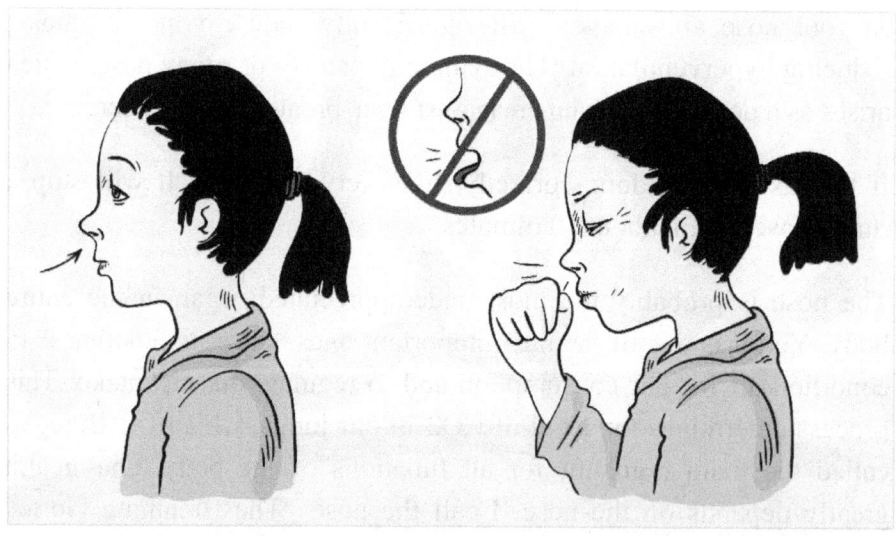

Chapter Eight

Peter's Mom's Journal

This is a story of a lifestyle change told by Helen, a client at Breathing Center whose son was afflicted with enlarged adenoids. She shared their story:

When I was told that Peter needs an adenoidectomy, I turned to the Internet and started searching for an alternative. About a month and a half ago, I discovered Breathing Normalization. We signed up for a course and since then our daily routine has changed drastically as we help Peter improve his breathing so he can recover his health.

On weekday mornings, I wake Peter up at 5:30, which is a half hour earlier than it used to be. This was difficult to adjust to at first, but it has been more than worth it, as we've watched his health improve. Breathing Normalization has affected every part of his life, from his mood, which is much better now, to his ability to focus in school. He's still sleepy when he first wakes up at this hour and as he goes to the bathroom and brushes his teeth. The adjustment period is over now, and after a full month of doing Breathing Normalization, Peter is really getting that this is an organic part of his routine, just as much as brushing his teeth is.

Once he's done in the bathroom, he comes back to his room, sits on a firm, wooden chair, and we measure his Control Pause together. He writes it in his logbook. Every day, we look at the logbook together, and it's great to see that his Control Pause has increased significantly—it was only 5 seconds when he started. Of course, there are ups and downs, but he's much more confident now. He's very aware of his progress and perceives it as success. He doesn't mind the perks either, because sometimes I get him a new toy as a reward for a significant increase in his Control Pause.

Next comes the jumping, running, walking exercise. At first, he had a hard time not talking, but now he gets that it's okay to talk between sets, but not during. Even the first set gets his blood flowing and he looks better right away. Sometimes, we don't have time to do all three sets, but I always try to create the time, even though it can be difficult for the whole family. Every set that he does brings him more calm, focus and clarity.

After he finishes the exercise, his breathing is deeper and more pronounced, which concerned me at the beginning. But then I learned that after the exercise he needs to sit down and rest for a few minutes until his breathing calms down.

Initially, I tried to get him to just sit there for 5 minutes, but it never worked because he was so revved up that he simply couldn't sit still. Then, I started using imagery to keep his mind occupied. I'd ask him to imagine his favorite soccer player, to imagine the ball, the field, details of his uniform, etc. This really relaxed him after a few minutes. Then, we both check to make sure his chest and stomach are barely moving and then we're done.

He showers, dresses and packs for school, which takes about 15 minutes—perfect, because we need to wait that long before measuring his post-session Control Pause. So, it's back to the firm chair, and we again measure his Control Pause. It's always exciting to see that it's higher than his Control Pause before the session.

Breakfast used to be a constant battle, a lengthy affair, because he didn't want to eat as much as I thought he should, and I would always insist. But since I learned that overeating is one of the causes of hyperventilation, I've completely changed my attitude about his appetite. And because we're no longer having the huge, filling dinners that we used to have, he's hungrier in the morning than he used to be. Also, if he does not want to eat dinner, I let him skip it. This has happened a few times now, and he then eats just about anything in the morning. Suddenly, he loves oatmeal when before he complained that it was too boring. No more bacon, his breakfast is mostly plant-based, with eggs once in a while. Portions are smaller now, and if he doesn't want to eat it all, I don't insist.

By the time Peter's done with breakfast, I have his lunch box ready to take to school. He used to eat the school cafeteria food, which is mostly heavily processed, but now I know that type of diet caused hyperventilation, so I pack a lunch for him. Usually, I make hearty soups with beans and vegetables or sandwiches with hummus and fresh vegetables. So instead of eating fries with chicken nuggets or a hot dog like he used to do, he eats healthy, organic food. Just thinking about it makes me feel good! Before, I was not aware that the food he used to eat at school contained all kinds of harmful chemicals, not to mention antibiotics and hormones. I would not say that this transition from "fun food everyone else is eating" to "healthy food just for him" was easy! Peter and I spent a lot of time talking about food, analyzing all the pros and cons of homemade organic food versus commercial food. We also watched a few documentaries on this topic. This is something we would have never done before we discovered Breathing Normalization. He now knows that chemical additives in food are a problem not only for people's health but also for the environment. On a more personal level, he understands that it makes his nose run. He doesn't eat junk food, not because he it's forbidden but because he understands the consequences of eating it.

Okay, back to our daily routine. Today is a chilly fall day and it used to be that I would always insist on Peter wearing a hat and a warm jacket. It was another point of contention because he never really wanted to, but I thought it was an essential step to keep him from catching a cold. And maybe it was, before his health started to improve so dramatically. But at this point, Peter's Control Pause is around 28 seconds, so it's safe, healthier actually, for him to be exposed to more extreme temperatures, because I now know that overheating is another cause of hyperventilation.

So today he doesn't want to wear a hat. He's picked out a sweater, but wants to wear shorts. I say, "Great! This way it's better for your health. I'm glad you feel healthy enough to wear this. I'm so proud of you! Maybe you can just take your jacket in your backpack in case you get cold later?" and he says, "Okay, sure, Mom."

This morning, Peter's dad is walking him to the school, something they both enjoy. We're lucky that the school is a twenty-minute walk from home because it's a great opportunity for some mild exercise and some breathing work as well. Sometimes, he plays the airplane game; sometimes, he does short breath holds, counting steps to time the holds and the space in between. Sometimes, he makes up a game with breath holds, which can get very silly, so he has fun with it.

At some point, I realized that I was neglecting Peter's health by working full-time and leaving him on his own so much. So I chose to go to a part-time schedule for three months, so I could really devote myself to helping him establish healthy breathing patterns. This is so important for Peter's health, not just now, but as a foundation for his life-long health. I feel strongly that this is my responsibility as his mother. Think about it: the best gift I can give my son for his future is perfect health, don't you think?

I know by Peter's Control Pause that his health is still not at 100 percent and that his energy level is still limited. So even though he's pretty hyper when he gets home from school, I know it's really important for him to rest. He doesn't realize that he's tired because he's so revved up, so it's on me to settle him down. I get him to sit with me on the couch and watch TV for 40 minutes. He likes to rest his head in my lap or have me put my arms around him. It makes him feel comfortable, safe, and relaxed. This is also a perfect opportunity to play with tape. Sometimes, I pretend that I forgot I have tape on my mouth and try to talk, which makes him laugh. He gets a kick out of my "forgetting." This time is a combination of rest, fun and breathing exercise for us, and after he's rested, relaxed and in a good mood.

I know by Peter's Control Pause that his health is still not at 100 percent and that his energy level is still limited. So even though he's pretty hyper when he gets home from school, I know it's really important for him to rest. He doesn't realize that he's tired because he's so revved up, so it's on me to settle him down. I get him to sit with me on the couch and watch TV for 40 minutes. He likes to rest his head in my lap or have me put my arms around him. It makes him feel comfortable, safe, and relaxed. This is also a perfect opportunity to play with tape. Sometimes, I pretend that I forgot I have tape on my mouth and try to talk, which makes him laugh. He gets a kick out of my "forgetting." This time is a combination of rest, fun and breathing exercise for us, and after he's rested, relaxed and in a good mood.

Peter used to have a full after-school schedule. Everything was timed down to the minute so we could cram it all in, but in learning about Breathing Normalization, I realized that he really was ill and that he didn't have enough energy for such a hectic schedule. So for now, his health is more important than any accomplishments. Once his breathing and his health are stronger, it won't be a problem for him to add back any extra-curricular activities he wants. Healthy breathing creates an oxygen-rich environment for the brain and supports focus and concentration. I know his capacities will increase tremendously and I'm already seeing the improvement. I'm very confident and hopeful, but for right now we've stopped most after-school activities for a three-month period, while he's working on his health. Now, he's got plenty of time to play with friends and play outside, take the dog for long walks, or do whatever he wants in the relaxing, unstructured time that he has.

Peter used to play soccer and tennis three times a week. Like many parents, we thought it was great for him, partly because those kind of activities help with getting into a good college. We didn't notice, at the time, that whenever he played tennis he always breathed through his mouth. He always ended up coughing a lot, didn't sleep well and turned moody and pale. Now we know that the strenuous physical activities triggered hyperventilation, and that if he couldn't breathe through his nose while playing sports, he needed to not participate in them for now. Peter loves tennis, so it was a disappointment for him, and for us, that he had to stop. But he can always come back to it in another month or so when he's healthy again. He is already able to run and breathe through his nose—something, which was impossible for him before. I am convinced that being able to breathe correctly and be healthy will only positively affect his athletic.

At first we were a little confused about this whole issue, because, obviously, he needs to be physically active, and with sports out of the picture, what were we going to replace them with? It's often rainy and grey here in New York in the fall, so our options are somewhat limited. We decided to get an Elliptical machine and were lucky to find a very good deal on Craigslist. Now, during homework time, he takes breaks on the machine. I started getting him audio versions of books he likes, so instead of sitting and reading, or playing video games, neither of which are good for his breathing, he can now listen to his favorite adventure books while he's exercising.

Before Breathing Normalization, our family dinners were probably typical for the average American family. We had meat just about every night, and when we didn't, we had cheesy pasta dishes. Peter's disease turned out to be a bit of a blessing for the whole family because it encouraged us to improve our diet. We no longer eat beef, pork and chicken every night—we've cut it down to two times a week and maybe fish once a week. Instead, we now generally eat simple, plant-based meals, organic whenever possible. Our dinners have become much more interesting because now I occasionally make ethnic food—Indian, Thai, or Mexican. Within this first month of "Peter's new diet" I lost eight pounds myself, which I'm very happy about!

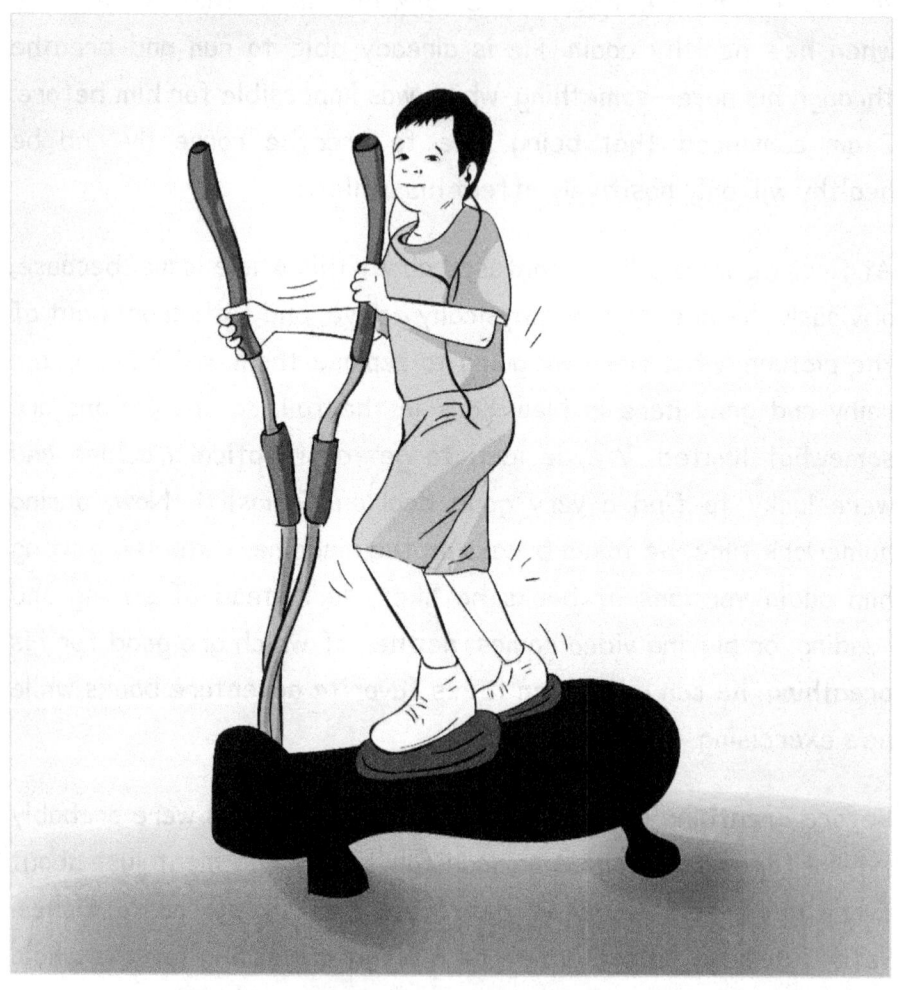

Tonight, I made steamed broccoli, brown rice with almonds with tahini sauce, and a big salad. Initially, we dreaded having to make this big of a change, but even my older daughter has been pleasantly surprised by how delicious good, healthy food can be. And since we're eating less processed foods and junk food, we all feel better and are generally in a better mood.

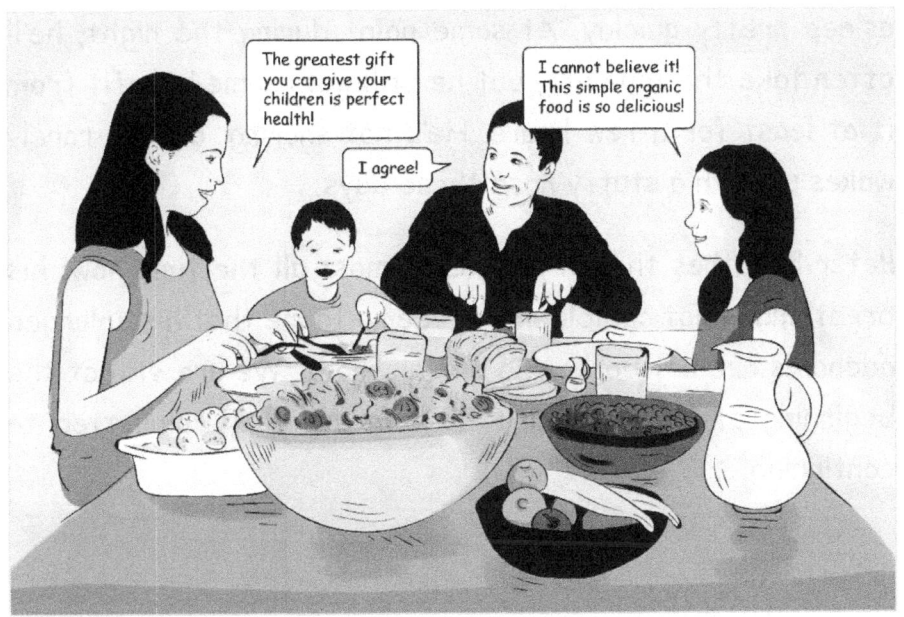

The whole family is trying to eat organic now. We're still not quite at 100%, but 80% is pretty good for us. At first, I thought buying so much organic food would be hard on the budget, but of course we're eating a lot less meat, so it has pretty much balanced out.

Dinner is fun because it's another opportunity for Peter to catch mom or dad mouth breathing, so we usually make sure to give him one or two chances. It always cracks him up, and he really likes that he's helping us with our breathing as we're helping him with his.

When it's bedtime, Peter's dad and I take turns sitting with Peter while he falls asleep. First, I help him tie his scarf around his rib cage, and then he tapes his mouth. We usually read to him while he does breath holds, and he normally falls asleep pretty quickly. At some point during the night, he'll often take the tape off, but he still gets some benefit from it at least for a few hours. He's not snoring, and he rarely wakes up with a stuffy nose these days.

Peter breathes though his nose almost all the time now; his breathing is not audible and it seems to me that his enlarged adenoids are not bothering him anymore. We are still at the beginning of our breathing training but fully committed to continuing.

Chapter Nine

Questions and Answers

Below are the most common questions parents ask a Breathing Normalization specialist and my answers to them.

Question: My son's adenoids are significantly larger than they should be. He catches colds and gets the flu often, and always has a runny nose and a cough. His doctor told us that adenoid surgery is unavoidable. Is there any alternative?

Answer: Years of clinical experience have shown that the Buteyko™ Breathing Normalization method helps children restore their breathing to norm. When a child stops over-breathing (especially mouth breathing), the adenoids not only stop obstructing nasal breathing, but in many cases shrink in size. At the same time, the immune system strengthens, and the child becomes less susceptible to colds or flu.

The typical hyperventilation symptoms of stuffy nose or cough gradually disappear as well. We suggest that you and your child start learning the Breathing Normalization method as soon as possible. We strongly urge you to continue seeing your child's physician. Only a medical professional can officially confirm that your child's adenoid condition has improved and that surgery is no longer necessary. You should consult an ENT for this diagnosis. Once this is taken care of, all you need to do is support your child in maintaining healthy nasal breathing.

Question: Do you suggest we reject the surgical removal of adenoids?

Answer: Absolutely not. Breathing Normalization specialists are not medical doctors; we are educators, and cannot make a decision about surgery. We teach children and their parents how to improve their breathing by eliminating hyperventilation (especially mouth breathing). Usually, this improves a child's health and removes all breathing difficulties, and as a result, the need for surgery is eliminated. However, this must be confirmed by a doctor. The final decision regarding surgery should be made by parents in consultation with their child's physician.

Question: How does the *Adenoids Without Surgery* program work?

Answer: For two months, a Breathing Normalization Specialist teaches the child to normalize his breathing through breathing exercises. The specialist also examines the child's lifestyle and makes recommendations to the parents on how to modify it so that it supports light nasal breathing. Everything in the program is adjusted to the individual student and his family. This typically helps the child avoid adenoidectomy, and significantly improves his respiratory, immune, nervous, and metabolic systems.

Answer: For two months, a Breathing Normalization Specialist teaches the child to normalize his breathing through breathing exercises. The specialist also examines the child's lifestyle and makes recommendations to the parents on how to modify it so that it supports light nasal breathing. Everything in the program is adjusted to the individual student and his family. This typically helps the child avoid adenoidectomy, and significantly improves his respiratory, immune, nervous, and metabolic systems.

Question: Adenoidectomy is not the only way to deal with adenoids. There are other options such as medication, laser treatment, acupuncture and homeopathy. How effective are they?

Answer: Those options can improve the condition of the adenoids, but if a child's over-breathing is not addressed, they will only bring temporary relief. Hyperventilation is what causes adenoids to become pathologically enlarged. To correct this situation in the long term, hyperventilation must be stopped.

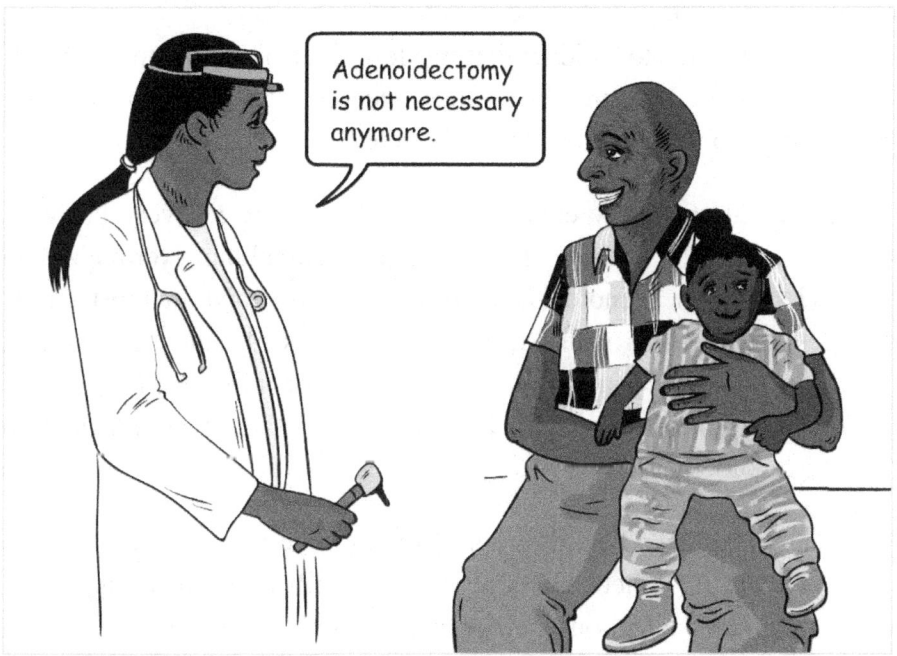

Question: My grandson does not sleep well at night because he cannot breathe through his nose. Will the Breathing Normalization method help? He does not have adenoid issues.

Answer: The Breathing Normalization method will help restore his nasal breathing and reduce his breathing to its norm. After his breathing is restored, most children start to sleep peacefully. We recommend you take our Breathing Normalization course right away because your grandson's current condition could lead to adenoid issues. If you address it now, it will prevent the development of more serious health issues such as enlarged adenoids, bronchitis or asthma.

Question: My son's adenoids have already been removed, but I've heard they can grow back. Will Breathing Center's work prevent the re-growth of adenoids?

Answer: Our experience demonstrates that breathing reduction prevents adenoids from growing back.

Question: The doctor told us that my four-year-old daughter needs an adenoidectomy. He said that if her adenoids are not removed, her health might become worse. Do you agree?

Answer: Pathologically enlarged adenoids can have a very negative effect on overall health. However, the Breathing Normalization method prevents adenoids from further growth, and in most cases, reduces their size as well. After a few months of Buteyko breathing exercises, doctors usually see a considerable improvement in the condition of the adenoids and often change their recommendation about adenoidectomies.

In some cases, the adenoids are already so large that it is necessary to remove them to protect one's health. It is still essential to apply the Breathing Normalization method right after the adenoidectomy to prevent the adenoids from growing back, otherwise the child may develop other health issues.

Question: I was told that enlarged adenoids could weaken a child's mental capacity. Should they be removed to prevent this?

Answer: It is not the adenoids, but hyperventilation that can damage brain development. To prevent this and other negative impacts of hyperventilation, the child's body creates a defense mechanism to make them breathe less—in this case, by enlarging the adenoids. It does not make sense to fight against this defense mechanism, but it is necessary to eliminate the root cause of the problem, which is over-breathing. The Breathing Center assists children and their parents in doing this.

Question: Are breathing exercises going to be difficult for my child?

Answer: Most children enjoy them as much as much as physical activities or games.

Question: How can I find a Breathing Normalization specialist to work with my child?

Answer: We will find a practitioner in your area or recommend one for you and your child to work with via Skype. Avoid working with unknown practitioners you find online, as they may not be certified by Breathing Center and Clinica Buteyko Moscow.

Question: My five-year-old daughter has enlarged adenoids. I want to take a Breathing Normalization program via Skype. What are the steps?

Answer: Your first step is to register for a Preliminary Consultation on our website: www.BreathingCenter.com. This will give you and your daughter an hour with an Advanced Breathing Normalization Specialist and a valuable overview of our program. If, after this consultation, you and the specialist are both convinced that the Breathing Normalization method will help your child, you can enroll in our Level 1 Breathing Normalization program, available in person and online.

Question: I am going to enroll in the Breathing Normalization program for my son, who is having issues with enlarged adenoids. But I am also concerned about my daughter, who seems to be developing asthma. Can my daughter attend the course as well? Will we have to pay the tuition twice?

Answer: Families can enroll in our Level 1 Breathing Normalization course as a group and pay only one tuition. All children are accompanied by a parent or guardian during their sessions, and the parent or guardian becomes the child's teacher and mentor outside of the formal sessions. We welcome other young family members to attend these sessions, or other adult family members who wish to support the primary student, or who have their own health issues they wish to address.

Question: I was told that I need to take the Level 1 program for my grandson with enlarged adenoids. Does that mean that we will then need to take Level 2?

Answer: No, the Level 1 program is sufficient for children with enlarged adenoids. Level 2 is an advanced program for adults only, and it is optional.

Question: I feel bad for children who have enlarged adenoids and want to help them. Can I become a Certified Breathing Normalization Specialist? If so, how?

Answer: You are welcome to take Level 1, 2 and 3 programs. All of them are available online, so you won't have to travel to Breathing Center. Upon completing the Level 3 program, you will receive a Breathing Normalization Specialist diploma and the rights to teach the method.

Question: I am trying to teach my daughter elements of the Breathing Normalization method, which I learned from a book and DVD. I am not sure that I am measuring her breathing correctly. I might be making other mistakes, too. What should I do?

Answer: Contact the Breathing Center and schedule a Private Session online with a Breathing Normalization Specialist. The Practitioner will check on how you work with your daughter's breathing and suggest corrections if necessary.

Chapter Ten

One More Testimonial

This is a story of a young client of mine who was very diligent in improving her breathing and health. She achieved good results greatly due to her parents' strong commitment.

A man from Dubai called me to ask if I could work with his daughter, Amrita. His daughter was very ill. Her adenoids had already been removed twice, but they grew back again. The day he called me, Amrita had visited her ENT doctor who informed her parents that their 6-year-old must have a third adenoidectomy.

Amrita was often sick, mostly with colds and flu, which were frequently treated with antibiotics. Antibiotics always stopped her symptoms, which made her parents hopeful, but after a while, her ailments would come back stronger. Her tonsils had bothered her, but not since they'd been treated with radiation. Amrita also suffered from periodic ear infections, which resulted in mild hearing loss. She was pale, sickly, and exhausted quickly. All these were typical signs of over-breathing.

I first met Amrita and her parents at our Preliminary Consultation online. Her Control Pause was only 3 seconds, which clearly indicated that this little girl was severely ill. She was a chronic mouth-breather. When I asked her to breathe through her nose, it seemed an impossible task. Of course, I knew that nasal breathing is always possible, but can be challenging for some kids with enlarged adenoids. It was also not easy for Amrita to stay focused. Because of her hindered hearing, she often asked me to repeat myself, which slowed our communication. Nevertheless, Amrita was cute and charming and extremely enthusiastic about her breathing training. Despite being severely ill, she was in high spirits.

Her parents were feeling desperate and willing to do anything to help their child. Conventional medical treatments had not helped, and by the time I met them, they were already fairly disillusioned with conventional treatment. In fact, within several years of them diligently following instructions from western doctors, Amrita's health became worse. At the same time, her parents were skeptical about alternative techniques and specifically about the Breathing Center, which they found on the Internet. But they did not have many options left. They decided to sign up for the Level 1 Breathing Normalization course, and I became their instructor.

I started seeing Amrita and her parents weekly via Skype and teaching them the Breathing Normalization method. To keep Amrita engaged and entertained, I often pretended to forget to breathe through my nose. She would immediately point it out and say, "Aunty Sasha, stop breathing through your mouth! It's bad for you!" Of course, this gave me the right to say the same back to Amrita. It took a few weeks to establish her nasal breathing during the day, but it was still loud. I remember asking Amrita to walk in place in front of the computer—she sounded like a small engine. "Amrita, I cannot believe it!" I would say. "Your breathing is so loud that I can even hear it in America!" That would get her attention; she would immediately notice her respiration and switch to quiet breathing. It was a pure pleasure to work with Amrita, who was very attentive and playful, even when the breathing games were not easy for her.

Amrita's mother told me that her daughter's breathing was quite alarming at night; she was, of course, breathing through her mouth and snored so loudly that it worried her parents. One night, they had recorded a video of Amrita while she slept and emailed me the recording. When I saw this video, I understood her parents' alarm. At night, this little darling girl turned into a monster, making wild, loud sounds with her wide-open mouth and then, all of a sudden, she would stop breathing. At the age of six, she had already developed sleep apnea.

When working with children, a lot depends on the parents. In Amrita's case, my work was fully supported by her father and mother, who participated in every session and started working on their own breathing. They created a true breathing improvement team, helping Amrita and each other. Her father joined a gym. Every morning before work, he would go there and do his workout, combined with breathing exercises. Her mother would do all the breathing exercises together with her daughter as her partner. At the beginning of our program, their breathing patterns were much better than their daughter's, yet by Dr. Buteyko's standards they were still far from optimal.

By modern medical standards, both parents were healthy except for allergies and some seasonal respiratory issues. Their first child, Amrita, was born healthy. As parents, they did their best for their daughter and yet she became ill, which puzzled them. Their younger son, who was a toddler at the time of our training, had already started hyperventilating. The parents wondered what was causing their children's poor health.

Both parents were from India, but a couple of years before we met, they had moved to Dubai. When I asked them about their childhoods, they told me they both grew up in rural India without much comfort. Meals were never left half-eaten and sometimes there were food shortages. Following Indian custom, both grew up as vegetarians. They ate mostly local, seasonal, and organic produce, not as a matter of choice, but simply because it was the only option. They lived in small houses, with all the kids sharing one or two rooms, and they spent a lot of time outside. When they were outdoors, they were usually barefoot and constantly in motion—playing with other kids or helping their parents.

They both said that they were both very healthy children. At that time, being ill was somewhat unusual. Sure, there were elderly people in bad health and people with various injuries, but Amrita's parents could not recall anyone among them who had frequent colds, flu, allergies, bronchitis or asthma. Most people were healthy where they grew up.

Both parents received educations; eventually, the father pursued a career and started making good money. Then, he met Amrita's mother; they got married and started their own family. Their life style changed drastically. They both admired a western lifestyle and wanted to provide the best for their children.

Amrita and her younger brother lived in a spacious and comfortable apartment. Amrita was driven everywhere in a car; she had many after-school activities, including swimming and aerobics classes. There was no need for her to spend time outside. Amrita had nice clothes, often made of synthetic fibers. Her parents purchased food at the supermarket and brought it home in plastic containers, frozen packages and cans. Amrita's lunch would often consist of a hotdog with French fries and a can of soda—food that would have been foreign to her parents when they were children and ate mostly rice, vegetables and fruits.

When Amrita was small, her parents believed in the power of western medicine. They did not understand the difference between Eastern and Western medical approaches: while Eastern doctors mostly try to find and eliminate the cause of disease, Western doctors mostly work with symptoms, suppressing or eliminating them. The first approach can be slow and cause discomfort because symptoms can remain active for as long as their cause is present. The second appears to be quick and effective since it provides the patient with immediate relief; however, in the long-term, it can actually damage health and generate more symptoms. Following the recommendations of Amrita's Western doctor, the parents were giving their daughter chemical drugs at the first signs of ailment. She also took antibiotics every year. When Amrita's breathing was compromised, she was told to use a rescue inhaler to increase the airflow to the lungs.

All in all, the parents' natural and simple lifestyle was discarded and a new, comfort-based, lifestyle was established. During my weekly sessions, I spent a significant time discussing and sharing ways to "undo it" by making simpler and more natural lifestyle choices. First, Amrita's parents resisted these alterations, mostly because they worked hard to provide their children with modern ways of living. This changed when they understood that too much comfort and an unnatural lifestyle can cause hyperventilation. They became eager to incorporate the changes. Fortunately, Amrita's father had a good sense of humor, making our discussions easier. I recommended the family stop using an expensive European toothpaste containing chemicals and switch to an Aurvedic powder made of over twenty healthful herbs. They were familiar with this tooth powder, which is common in India. "Well, we use Indian products only if someone from America recommends them," Amrita's father joked.

During the course of our Breathing Normalization program, Amrita's parents made significant dietary changes. They went back to being vegetarian and found a source for fresh, organic produce in Dubai. They started eating food free of harmful chemicals and genetic modification. It was not easy for them to let their children play outside, mostly due to a lack of time as well as Dubai's unbearably hot summers, but where there's a will there's a way.

They invited Amrita's grandmother to stay with them and help with the kids. The grandmother would get up at sunrise and take Amrita and her little brother to the seaside while the air was cool. Amrita enjoyed running barefoot on the sand, splashing in the sea, and collecting pretty stones. It was rejuvenating for both children just as much as it was for their grandmother and their parents, who occasionally joined them.

When Amrita's mother was young, she studied martial arts and had a Black Belt in Karate. This took diligence and discipline—qualities that are also essential for Breathing Normalization. It did not take long for Amrita's mother to realize she possessed something precious that she could pass on to her daughter. She started treating Amrita's daily breathing sessions the same way she used to treat her martial arts training. Missing a session was not an option; breathing games were treated seriously and with respect. This not only helped improve Amrita's breathing but also strengthened their bond. Amrita also learned how to set a goal and achieve it though diligence and hard work.

It pleased Amrita's parents to see that their daughter was getting healthier every week. Nevertheless, she still had some respiratory problems. At one point, her parents discovered that there was a conflict between the medication prescribed to Amrita by her ENT and her breathing training. The purpose of the breathing training was to reduce breathing by making it gentler and lighter while some medications triggered hyperventilation.

It was not my place to pass judgment about the recommendations of Amrita's doctor; however, I encouraged the parents to learn everything they could about the medication they were giving their six-year-old. They read the small print and did research online. It was shocking for them to discover that Amrita's drugs came with serious side effects, which could negatively impact various organs and bodily systems, including their daughter's respiratory system. While we were working on Amrita's breathing improvement, the medications she was taking were often in opposition to the goals we were working towards. Eventually, Amrita's parents decided that it was time to make a change. They found a good Ayurvedic doctor in Dubai who supported Amrita's health normalization process.

This decision accelerated Amrita's progress. Being supported by the healing power of herbs, her remaining symptoms disappeared, and she regained a strong respiratory system and full health Nonetheless, I advised her parents to continue seeing an ENT to check on the size of Amrita's adenoids and her respiratory health. Three months after the beginning of our breathing training, her doctor said that an adenoidectomy was no longer necessary.

Even without his diagnosis, it was easy to see that Amrita's adenoids stopped bothering her. She was breathing through her nose all the time—while still or in motion, awake or asleep, silent or talking. Her breathing was quiet and invisible, the way healthy breathing is supposed to be. Amrita's face regained color; she became energetic but calmer; she no longer snored or experienced sleep apnea; her nose, which used to be congested, was now clear. The dry cough, which had bothered Amrita, had also disappeared. Even her hearing was restored, which is a known result of Breathing Normalization. Her tonsils and adenoids were no longer an issue. Her adenoids did not disappear but they shrank significantly, since the swelling of the mucus membrane was gone. They stopped obstructing Amrita's breathing. If she continues breathing through her nose, I'm sure they would atrophy within a few years.

Amrita successfully completed the Level 1 course and became healthy. To solidify these changes into their lives, her parents had to continue with their healthy lifestyle and new breathing habits. This shouldn't be a difficult task: maintaining healthy breathing patterns is much easier than establishing them. As a result of Amrita's training, both parents also became healthier and more energetic. They also learned how to take care of their younger son to prevent health difficulties like they had with Amrita.

The only problem they experienced with their six-year-old daughter was Amrita's attitude toward breathing at the end of our program. She would catch her friends, relatives and even teachers breathing through their mouth and immediately say, "Stop breathing through your mouth! It is bad for your health! Believe me, I know!" After that, she would demonstrate her 80 second Positive Maximum Pause and challenge the person to measure his or hers and evaluate the state of their breathing and health. Obviously, she loved pretending to be a Breathing Normalization specialist!

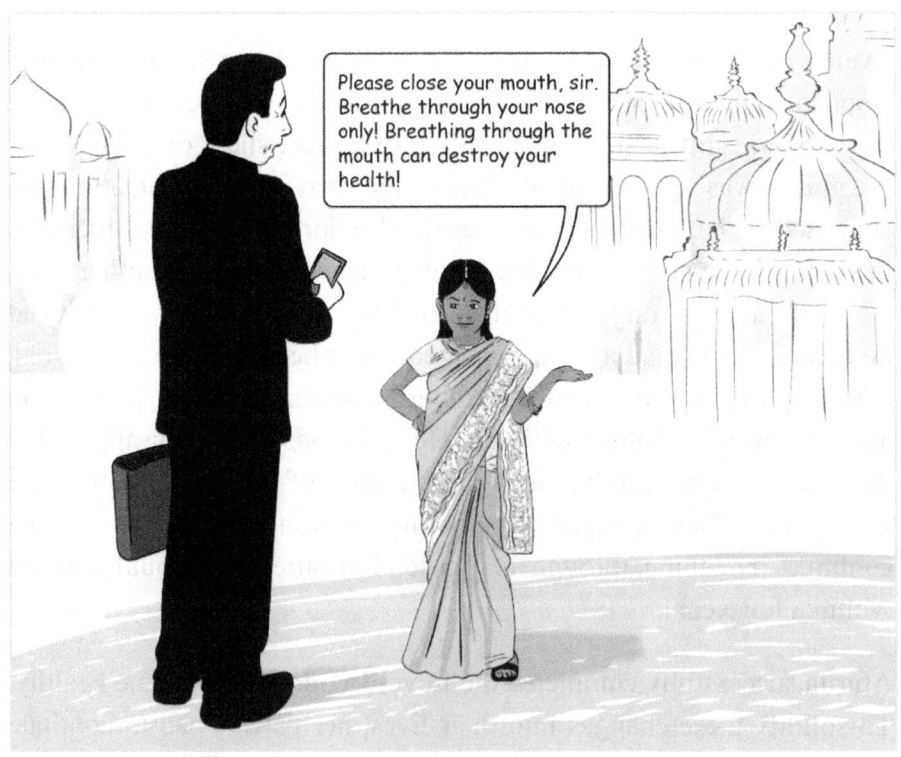

Breathing Logbook

How to use this logbook:

To apply the Breathing Normalization method correctly, a student needs to document breathing measurements. This chapter will help you accomplish this task. Use this logbook to record your child's progress as well as your own.

I recommend that a child do three formal sessions of breathing exercises every day, preferably in the morning, the middle of the day and before going to bed. Each session of formal breathing exercises should be about 30 minutes long (it can be shorter, but preferably, not longer).

Every seated session starts with relaxation and continues with breath holds or other types of exercises suitable for a formal session.

A recording of guided relaxation techniques, which are called *Breathing Normalization Meditations*, is available as a free download on the Breathing Center's website. These meditations are helpful for both children and adults. If it is a session in motion, relaxation could be skipped.

To determine the appropriate length of breath holds, please follow the instructions in this book or consult with a Breathing Normalization specialist.

To record your child's breathing data, you will need to measure his Control Pause (CP) or his Positive Maximum Pause (PMP). Usually, students measure their CP in the beginning of their training and switch to measuring PMP when CP becomes stable on the level above 20 seconds. To understand how to measure CP/PMP, please follow the instructions in this book or visit the *Self-Test page* of Breathing Center's website or watch the 1st disc of the DVD, *The Breathing Normalization Method,* available as a download from the same website—**www.BreathingCenter.com**

What measurements to record in this logbook?

1. **Morning CP or PMP**: Each morning, measure your child's CP or PMP. This is the most important data of the day, which reflects significant shifts in his habitual breathing patterns.

2. **Before and After CP or PMP**: Measure your child's CP/PMP before and after each formal session of breathing exercises. This will help to ensure that your child is doing the exercises correctly. If his CP/PMP is higher after doing the exercises, then he has done them successfully. Conversely, if his CP or PMP is lower after doing the breathing exercises, then he has done them incorrectly.

3. **Type of Breathing Exercises**: make notes of what exercises have been done during each session. For example, relaxation (Relax), breath holds (BHs), Three-Fold Jumps (3FJ), or other types. If a child does breath holds, I recommend recording their length.

Example of Log Recordings on following page.

Breathing Logbook

DATE/ DAY	MORNING CP/PAIP	BEFORE CP/PAIP	1st SESSION	AFTER CP/PAIP	BEFORE CP/PAIP	2nd SESSION	AFTER CP/PAIP	BEFORE CP/PAIP	3rd SESSION	AFTER CP/PAIP
2/26 Tues.	CP: 3 sec.	CP: 5 sec.	30 min: Relax+BHs Fixed BHs: 4 sec.	CP: 7 sec.	CP: 4 sec.	20 min.: Relax+BHs fixed BHs: 3 sec.	CP: 4 sec.	CP: 5 sec.	30 min: Relax+BHs Flexible BHs: 3-6 sec.	CP: 8 sec.
2/27 Weds.	CP: 5 sec.	CP: 6 sec.	30 min: Relax+BHs Flexible BHs: 3-8 sec.	CP: 9 sec.	CP: 7 sec.	10 min: just BHs Flexible: 6-9 sec.	CP: 6 sec.	CP: 5 sec.	30 min: Relax+BHs Fixed BHs: 5 sec.	CP: 7 sec.
2/28 Thur.										
2/29 Fri.										
2/30 Sat.										

Breathing Logbook

DATE/DAY	MORNING CP/PAP	BEFORE CP/PAP	1st SESSION	AFTER CP/PAP	BEFORE CP/PAP	2nd SESSION	AFTER CP/PAP	BEFORE CP/PAP	3rd SESSION	AFTER CP/PAP

Afterword

By Ira J Packman, MD

Since turning 65 years old, I have been reflecting on my career as a "healer." After internal medicine training, I found myself in Northwest New Mexico, where I started a multispecialty group with two other physicians and a physician assistant from my training program in Harrisburg, Pennsylvania. In New Mexico, I was exposed to many healers—alternative practitioners and health educators, including medicine men from many Native American tribes, herbalists and acupuncturists. After I moved back to Harrisburg, I continued to utilize the teachings and practices of healers in the care of my patients.

My practice was very traditional in the sense that we all trained as medical doctors in medical schools. Along with my partners, whom I had known since medical school, we grew into a very large internal medicine group and were *hospitalists* before the term even existed. We were all board certified in internal medicine and ended up seeing very sick patients in the ICU/CCU—at times caring for close to 100 patients a day in the hospital setting. It was not unusual for us to spend 12-16 hours a day in the hospital. For the past ten years, I have been a consultant to the State of Pennsylvania for "Standard of Care."

I only go into this detail so the reader of this Afterword understands that I am a very traditionally (allopathically-MD) trained internist. I have used practitioners in many of the healing arts for over forty years to help my patients. During the thirty-four years I was in clinical practice, I frequently referred patients to Chiropractors, Homeopathic Physicians, Massage Therapists, Podiatrists, Acupuncturists, Herbalists, Naturalists, Physical Therapists and to Breathing

Afterword by Ira J Packman, MD

Normalization specialists at the Breathing Center, who taught the Buteyko Breathing Normalization method which is described in this book.

After I met Sasha Yakovleva and her husband, Thomas Fredricksen, co-founders of the Breathing Center, and I was introduced to the Breathing Normalization method, I read much of Dr. K. P. Buteyko's research and watched some of his original patient films. I have also had the privilege of speaking directly with Dr. A. E. Novozhilov, the stepson of Dr. Buteyko, who worked side by side with Dr. Buteyko for years. My involvement with the Buteyko Method has made me think very differently about the origin of many diseases.

Dr. Buteyko's original work, and the subsequent work carried on by Dr. Novozhilov, challenges the very core of what most Allopathic-M.D. or Osteopathic-D.O. physicians believe is the basis of many diseases. This is not dissimilar to the challenge encountered by Samuel Hahnemann at the end of the 18th century, when he first described the principles of homeopathy. The premise that *"illness is the expression of self-healing"* is the basis of homeopathy, and is totally applicable to the Buteyko Method and explanation of disease. Hahnemann talked about the "vital force" and "power of recovery" and described a principal of *"Similars."* In the traditional homeopathic process, physicians determined each healthy individual's response or set of symptoms when exposed to every natural element available. When that person became ill, they would give a small dose of the *"same"* element which caused the symptoms that were now present. They would see an exaggeration of the symptoms (curative response) and then the symptoms would fade away (just as Sasha describes in the part of this book about the Healing Crisis). **It was a deficiency in that natural element that caused the symptoms.** *Replace the deficient element and the patient gets better.*

In Buteyko theory, *the element which is deficient is carbon dioxide (CO_2).* This element is chronically deficient because of persistent hyperventilation. Chronic hyperventilation is a very slight, almost imperceptible increase in the depth and rate of breathing. This causes the lungs to expel too much CO_2, which immediately raises the body's pH. In response to this elevated pH, the body tries to correct the problem with "compensatory mechanisms." The kidneys decrease their excretion of CO_2 by reabsorbing CO_2 from the urine. This causes an increase in the excretion of positively charged minerals, including calcium (Ca), magnesium (Mg) and phosphorous (P) because they are linked to the reabsorption of CO_2. The loss of phosphorous (P), lowers the body's stores of ATP (the energy molecule), which compromises many organ systems. This subsequently affects muscle contraction, muscle fatigue and nerve conduction of electrical impulses. In an attempt to retain CO_2 in the lungs, the airways in the lungs constrict, causing wheezing, and the adenoids swell to try to decrease the CO_2 being expelled with each breath.

Hyperventilation
(The primary disease)
↓
CO2 loss from the lungs
↓
Increase body's pH acutely—and chronically)
↓   ↓

Kidneys retain CO2 and lose positively charged elements (Mg, CA, P, K)   **The upper airways change to restrict the outgoing flow of CO2 (Wheezing, adenoids enlarge)**

Patients develop enlarged adenoids, asthma, hypertension, immune deficiency, allergies, many other diseases.

Afterword by Ira J Packman, MD

This goes against everything we are taught as allopathically trained physicians. *Hyperventilation is the primary disease process. Asthma and adenoid enlargement are the bodies normal compensatory mechanisms (the "expressions of self-healing") which occur as the body tries to correct the abnormal pH created by the chronic hyperventilation.*

Note to all of you traditionally trained medical practitioners: think about this concept before dismissing it just because it is not what you were taught and you don't understand it. *Know that Buteyko Breathing Normalization method works*—it works dramatically. Patients get better! This is as revolutionary as when Einstein told us that $E=MC^2$. It is a total restructuring of the primary cause of many diseases.

Of all healers I have met while practicing medicine for thirty-four years, Sasha Yakovleva is one of those people who truly understands the concept of helping patients. She can guide you and your children to a truly healthy state and help you attain balance of Mind, Body and Spirit, which is the definition of "Health." Even though as a Breathing Normalization specialist, Sasha was trained by doctors in Clinica Buteyko Moscow, I call her "Healer" because she has a talent to heal people through health education.

In this amazing book, Sasha has written a guide for all people to improve their health by establishing the best breathing patterns possible. Although this book is targeted for children with enlarged adenoids, all children—as well as parents—who engage in Breathing Normalization will become healthier, stronger, more balanced and more content.

On the surface, the content of this book appears very simple. Do not let the simplicity of the contents of this book fool you. Sasha tells me that Dr. Buteyko always said that "his method is very simple, but its application is not." That is very true. Sasha is a healer, health educator and teacher. If you follow her instructions, do the exercises and implement the life style changes, you and your children will feel better and be healthier and more balanced. Read her book, do the exercises, make the changes.

Ira J Packman M.D.

Harrisburg, PA 2015

March 5, 2015

About the Author and Contributors

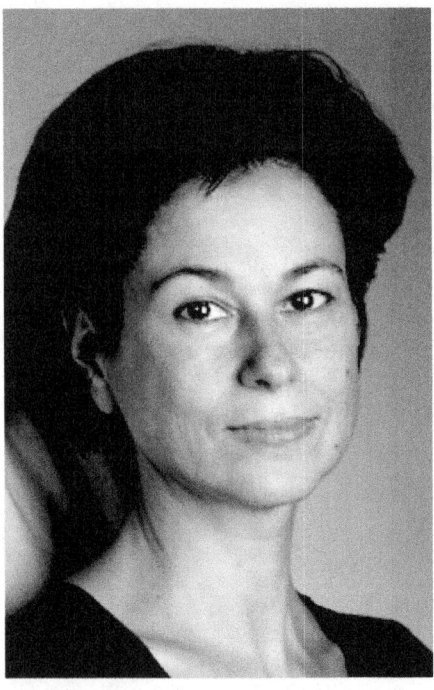

Sasha Yakovleva is an Advanced Breathing Normalization Specialist and co-founder of BreathingCenter.com in the USA.

She first came across Dr. Buteyko's approach while searching for natural methods to combat her husband's severe asthma. The Buteyko™ method helped him overcome his disease and become healthy. It also helped Sasha to stop her health problems such as sleep apnea, allergies, kidney and joints problems. Sasha received her training from A. Novozhilov MD and other doctors at Clinica Buteyko in Moscow as well as Dr. Buteyko's widow.

Sasha holds a Master Degree in Journalism. She studied holistic techniques around the world and has written about them extensively for over twenty-five years. Originally from Russia, in 1990 Sasha started publishing the first Russian holistic magazine, which became a large national publication. Soon after, she opened the first health food store in Moscow. She wrote the book, *Anthology of Inward Path*, containing many articles and interviews with healers, progressive scientists, doctors and spiritual leaders from Russia and other countries. She traveled extensively in Asia, Europe and America, researching and writing about various *mind, body, and spirit* modalities.

Since 1993, Sasha has been practicing various forms of meditation under the guidance of Tibetan Buddhist lamas. She completed several short and long periods of intense practice.

For the last fifteen years, she has been residing in the US. Currently, she lives in Colorado mountains near Boulder. As a Breathing Normalization specialist, she works with adults and children around the world. She is the Executive Director of BreathingCenter.com, which officially represents Dr. Buteyko's work outside Russia.

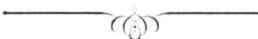

Ira Packman, MD wrote the afterword for this book. He is a member of the American Medical Association, a Board certified Internal Medicine Physician, and presently a Medical consultant to the State of Pennsylvania on Standard of Care. As a life-long asthmatic, Dr. Packman tried every approach available to overcome his breathing difficulties. He was able to significantly improve his condition by applying the Breathing Normalization method. Dr. Packman firmly believes in this method. He lives and works in Pennsylvania.

This book is illustrated by **Arash Akhgari**. As a child growing up in Iran, Arash experienced breathing difficulties due to his enlarged adenoids, which eventually were surgically removed. Coming across Breathing Center's work helped him to realize the danger of hyperventilation and start improving his breathing. His drawings helped many Breathing Center's students—parents and especially children—to avoid adenoidectomy and become healthier. Arash lives in Canada.

And last, but not least, we want to acknowledge the **parents** who took the Breathing Normalization programs at the Breathing Center to help their children prevent an adenoidectomy. Two chapters in this book are written by them.

Made in United States
North Haven, CT
22 December 2023